The Overflowing Brain

The Overflowing Brain
Information Overload and the
Limits of Working Memory

Torkel Klingberg, MD, PhD

Professor of Cognitive Neuroscience
Karolinska Institute
Stockholm Brain Institute
Stockholm, Sweden

Translated by Neil Betteridge

OXFORD
UNIVERSITY PRESS

2009

OXFORD
UNIVERSITY PRESS

Oxford University Press, Inc., publishes works that further
Oxford University's objective of excellence
in research, scholarship, and education.

Oxford   New York
Auckland   Cape Town   Dar es Salaam   Hong Kong   Karachi
Kuala Lumpur   Madrid   Melbourne   Mexico City   Nairobi
New Delhi   Shanghai   Taipei   Toronto

With offices in
Argentina   Austria   Brazil   Chile   Czech Republic   France   Greece
Guatemala   Hungary   Italy   Japan   Poland   Portugal   Singapore
South Korea   Switzerland   Thailand   Turkey   Ukraine   Vietnam

Published by Oxford University Press, Inc.
198 Madison Avenue, New York, New York 10016
www.oup.com

Oxford is a registered trademark of Oxford University Press

Library of Congress Cataloging-in-Publication Data

Klingberg, Torkel, 1967-
[Översvämmade hjärnan]
The overflowing brain: information overload and the limits of working
memory / Torkel Klingberg.
p. ; cm.
Includes bibliographical references and index.
ISBN: 978-0-19-537288-5
1.   Human information processing—Physiological aspects. 2.   Short-term
memory—Physiological aspects. 3.   Attention—Physiological aspects.
4.   Cerebral cortex—Growth. 5.   Neuroplasticity. I. Title.
[DNLM: 1.   Memory. 2.   Attention. 3.   Memory Disorders—pathology.
4.   Neuronal Plasticity—physiology. BF 371 K654o 2009]
BF444. K5513 2009
153—dc22
2008014273

Printed in the United States of America
on acid-free paper

To Hannah and Linnea

ACKNOWLEDGMENTS ■

I would like to thank all my friends and colleagues who have read, commented upon, and discussed the early drafts of this book. Thanks also to Tobias Nordqvist, my editor at Natur och Kultur, who gave me much constructive feedback, and Lena Forssén and Lotte Mjöberg at Natur och Kultur. Jan-Eric Gustafsson and Magnus Enquist provided valuable comments on the sections on intelligence and evolution, respectively.

For the English translation of the book I am grateful of the excellent work of Neil Betteridge. I would like to thank Elkhonon Goldberg for his kind foreword, and to the people at Oxford University Press who helped with the English edition: Craig Panner, David D'Addona, and Sue Warga.

Finally, thanks to my mother and father, to Anna-Karin for all the support, and to Hannah and Linnea for the inspiration they give me.

Foreword ■

Midtown Manhattan has never been a tranquil place, but over the last decade or so its rhythm has reached a new level of frenzy. Cell phones and iPods have arrived with a vengeance! Have they provided the inflexion point on society's path to self-destruction? People are listening, talking, texting, taking pictures, all while trying not to bump into one another with mixed success. It is an everyday occurrence to see people tripping over one another, over inanimate objects, over dogs, stumbling, slipping, falling, bumping into walls, nearly run over by cars—while clinging to their cell phones.

While the image of a befuddled pedestrian exceeding his or her capacity for multitasking by having one gadget too many can be hilarious, it is emblematic of our times and of the general challenges facing our culture. We are increasingly driven by information flows, and while politicians and economists worry about an insufficient flow of oil to keep our society going, we should be equally concerned about an increasingly excessive and overlapping flow of information that leaves the average member of our species increasingly distracted and disoriented.

How much multitasking can an average human being engage in without being run over by a car or by a fellow citizen? Has our culture reached, or perhaps exceeded, the capacity of the brain, which evolved from a far more sedate world? Are there limits to the human capacity for multi-tasking and for parallel processing? Can these limits be rigorously studied? Can they be expanded by training our brains?

Very few people are in a better position to address these questions than Torkel Klingberg. Dr. Klingberg has studied and conducted important research both in Sweden and in the United States, and he stands out among his colleagues by his ability to combine cutting-edge basic research in cognitive neuroscience with an eye for the potential of the results for patients and in every day life. Dr. Klingberg is Professor of Cognitive Neuroscience at the famed Karolinska Institute in Stockholm, where he spearheads a large research program using state-of-the-art technologies like functional magnetic resonance imaging (fMRI) and diffusion tensor imaging (DTI), as well as neural-network modeling, to elucidate the mechanisms of executive functions, attention, and of the various ways in which they may become aberrant in development. His research has also resulted in a method for cognitive rehabilitation through training of working memory, a method now in use both in Europe and the United States.

The brain is very much in vogue. Over the last few years popular books about the brain have become a literary genre in and of itself. *The Overflowing Brain* stands out among these books owing to its breadth, lucidity, and to its engaging narrative. The book first appeared in Swedish in 2007 and was met with great success. This is the first general-interest book in English which covers a comparable range of topics at a comparably authoritative level and with a comparable quality of writing. This makes the English-language edition of *The Overflowing Brain* particularly welcome and timely.

With effortless virtuosity, Klingberg interweaves the discussion of evolution, history of neuroscience, cutting-edge research methodologies, information theory, recent insights into neuroplasticity, and a thoughtful review of various neurodevelopmental disorders in order to better explain our "overflowing brain." While many of the "brain books" for the general public are written by professional journalists and science writers purveying second-hand knowledge of cognitive neuroscience, Klingberg's book is authoritative, having the advantage of being written by a true leader of the field. Klingberg does not pull any punches: He gives the reader the proper respect by being precise and substantive, without diluting the narrative with vacuous cuticisms so common, unfortunately, in "trade books." At the same time, what makes *The Overflowing Brain* particularly remarkable is its literary seamlessness that would make a professional science writer proud. This unique combination of substance and form will make the book valuable both for the educated general public as a high-level "trade book," and for the professional audience, perhaps even as a secondary text for students.

Like most fields of human endeavor, cognitive neuroscience and clinical neuropsychology has its fads. As is often the case, trendy notions rapidly become diffuse, opaque, inflated, and devoid of clear content. "Working memory" was a pioneering concept introduced by leading neuroscientists like Alan Baddeley and Patricia Goldman-Rakic, but it has since become a fad with all the untoward consequences thereof. Klingberg makes a particularly valuable contribution by restoring scientific rigor and clarity to the concept of "working memory." This is one of the many qualities that make *The Overflowing Brain* invaluable both for the general public and for the professional audience.

Attention Deficit Hyperactivity Disorder (ADHD) is another example of an originally valuable and meaningful concept having been diluted and inflated beyond recognition, scientific merit, or clinical legitimacy. Here, too, Klingberg provides an invaluable service both to the profession and to the general public by judiciously rendering ADHD with admirable rigor and clarity.

It has been said that "familiarity breeds contempt." Familiarity also breeds the illusion of understanding. The notion of Intelligence Quotient (IQ) has been part of the mainstream culture for so long that it is common among the members of the general public to invoke it with the casual aura of comprehension. In reality, however, very few members of the general public can offer an accurate definition of IQ if asked. Klingberg does a marvelous job explaining it and putting it into a rigorous neuroscientific and social-scientific context.

The Overflowing Brain is rich in insights and information—too many to review them all in this brief introduction. This is a truly remarkable book that will be read and enjoyed by members of the general public and the professional audience alike.

Elkhonon Goldberg
New York
May 2008

CONTENTS ■

THE OVERFLOWING BRAIN

1 ■

Introduction: The Stone Age Brain
Meets the Information Flood

You've just entered a room, probably to fetch something, but you're not that sure, for you're staring at the wall trying to remember what it was you were going to do. The instruction to yourself that you had in your head only a moment ago has vanished. Maybe you were distracted by your cell phone? Perhaps you were trying to do two or three things at the same time? Whatever, the outcome was a surplus of information in your brain that left you standing there gazing blankly at the wall.

Our brains have limited capacity for processing information. This book is an attempt to understand why this is so, what effect it has on our everyday lives, and how we can stretch these limits with mental exercise.

As advances in information technology and communication supply us with information at an ever accelerating rate, the limitations of our brains become all the more obvious. Boundaries are defined no longer by technology but by our own biology. These developments are particularly noticeable in our increasingly complex offices. Let us, by way of example, consider Linda, a fictional person who's nonetheless based on a close friend of mine and who has a work situation that will no doubt be familiar to many of us.

Linda is project manager at an IT company. Her Monday mornings start at half past eight as she seats herself at her desk in her open-plan office. With her cup of coffee at her side, she starts going through the weekend's crop of e-mails. She decides which are to be dumped, which are to be read but not dealt with, which should be responded to immediately, and which will end up as yet another item on her to-do list, which she updates and reprioritizes on her PC and then synchronizes with her BlackBerry. Come ten o'clock, she still hasn't got through her e-mails but decides to tackle the first item on her to-do list: write a report and read through four of her employees' progress reports. Three minutes into her report, she gets interrupted by a colleague who needs the go-ahead on a computer purchase. They log on to the computer company's Web site to take a quick look at the options available, but they're interrupted by a phone call to Linda about an e-mail from last Friday. The call goes on and on, and her colleague returns to his desk while Linda tries to ignore the signals from her cell phone as she frantically searches for the e-mail that the call's about. As she listens she takes the opportunity, while she has the e-mail program up, to delete some spam.

Thus the modern office. A survey of workplaces in the United States found that the personnel were interrupted and distracted roughly every three minutes and that people working on a computer had on average eight windows open at the same time. In his article "Overloaded Circuits: Why Smart People Underperform," psychiatrist Edward Hallowell coins the term "attention deficit trait" to characterize the situation in which Linda and many others find themselves. This is not a new diagnosis of any use to doctors, but rather a description of the mental state that information technology, a faster pace, and changing work patterns have induced. Some would call it a lifestyle. But the term "attention deficit trait" has been chosen for its similarity with the term "attention deficit disorder" (ADD), which is a variant of attention deficit hyperactivity disorder (ADHD) without the hyperactivity (more about ADHD later). The diagnosis is defined by a string of symptoms such as "difficulty sustaining attention," "difficulty organizing tasks or activities," "easily distracted by extraneous stimuli," and "forgetful in daily activities." Often these difficulties are so serious that they prevent people from doing their jobs properly or require medication. The point of Hallowell's term is that it illustrates how the modern work situation, with its pace and simultaneous demands, often gives us the feeling of having attention difficulties and of not quite having the capacity to do our jobs. Our brains are being flooded. But is it really the case that the information society generally impairs people's attentional abilities? What *are* attentional abilities, anyway, and exactly what in our complex work situations is mentally demanding?

One demand factor in our working lives is the incessant distractions: all the impressions that buzz around us like mosquitoes and make it hard for us to concentrate on what we're doing. The torrent of information increases not only the volume of data we're expected to take in but also the volume we need to shut out. One example of a change in the degree of distraction is in the transformation of a traditional office into an open-plan one. Such a rearrangement might improve communication between employees and be more stimulating, but it also gives us a greater influx of impressions in the shape of ringing phones, chatter, and SMS signals that we have to try to ignore. Another example of increasing demands is the way we source more and more information from the Internet instead of books or newspapers. It's usually perfectly possible to read an article in a newspaper without being distracted by advertisements in the margin; reading articles on the Internet, their margins packed with little animated advertisements, presents more of a challenge, however. What is it in our brains that determines whether we can concentrate and ignore the distractions?

Multitasking is the quick and easy solution for all those who want to get more done in less time. However, doing (or at least trying to do) several tasks simultaneously is one of our most demanding everyday activities. Running on a treadmill while watching TV usually isn't too taxing, nor is chewing gum while walking in a straight line. But even such a mundane situation as talking on a cell phone while driving is not as easy as we'd like to think. Apart from the fact that it's difficult to hold the wheel and shift gears with the same hand, or to keep our eyes on the road and on the phone's display at the same time, there's something in the mentally demanding task of telephoning that makes us worse drivers. Tests show that people who drive while performing a mentally demanding task have a reaction time that is up to one and a half seconds slower. Why can't we combine some activities with others? Why is the brain sometimes unable to do two things at once?

The issue of simultaneous performance is particularly interesting right now, as technological progress seems to encourage or indeed even require it. Thanks to the wireless revolution, we can take technology pretty much anywhere we want to. We chat on the phone while walking, driving, or watching television. We can have little displays in our cars showing maps that are continually updated and direct us as we drive. While in meetings we can text people or read e-mails on our BlackBerry. When the day is done and we're sitting in front of our television, a simultaneous scrolling line of text feeds us with extra information; some TV sets let us watch one channel inserted into another. We can sit on the sofa with our laptop while watching television, wirelessly connected to the Internet.

Our relationship to information is ambivalent. We clearly often seek out more, quicker, and more complex information, as if we're getting a kick from the shot. But when we're sitting on the sofa trying to read the on-screen text while trying to follow the headlines, many of us are struck with a feeling of inadequacy, with a sense that our brain is already full of information. It's overflowing.

New findings in psychology and brain research suggest that the difficulties we find with simultaneous performance and distractions converge onto one central limitation: the ability to retain information. When you're trying to do two things at once, you have to juggle two different sets of instructions in your head. This is double the amount of information relative to if you only had one instruction. When you're distracted, you often end up losing the original information, which leaves you standing in a room without knowing what you're doing there.

Our limited ability to retain information can be illustrated with two situations in which the volume of information increases. If you're given directions of the "Go straight ahead for two blocks and then left one block" kind, you'll probably have no trouble remembering them. However, if the description is more like "Go straight ahead for two blocks and then one block to the left and the right again for three blocks, then left and then three right, and you're there," your chances of getting lost start to increase. It is too much information. Similarly, a four-digit PIN is quite easy to remember once you've heard it, but a twelve-digit OCR code is almost impossible to keep in your head.

■ The Magical Number Seven

"My problem, ladies and gentlemen, is that I have been persecuted by an integer." Thus began George Miller in his 1956 article "The Magical Number Seven, Plus or Minus Two: Some Limits on Our Capacity for Processing Information." The hypothesis contained within is that there is a fixed capacity for the human ability to receive information, and that this limit lies at around seven items. There is, in other words, an inherent constraint on the brain's bandwidth. The article proved to be one of the most influential in twentieth-century psychology.

By the mid-1950s, when Miller wrote his article, there was a surge in interest in the term *information* in psychology. Scientists had started developing computers during World War II to help them crack enemy codes. Mathematicians and physicists proposed ways of quantifying the concept of information and examining the limitations of conveying information on the phone down copper wires from one person to another. Miller's idea was that psychologists could look at the human brain in exactly the same way as physicists looked at copper wires. The brain was a "communication channel" of measurable speed, not unlike Internet hookups that let only a certain amount of information through per unit of time.

The crux of Miller's article is that there are limits to our brain's capacity. The number seven, he points out, pops up with uncanny frequency and has the power to stimulate the imagination, as Miller describes at the end: "What about the seven wonders of the world, the seven seas, the seven deadly sins, the seven daughters of Atlas in the Pleiades, the seven ages of man, the seven levels of hell, the seven primary colours, the seven notes of the musical scale, and the seven days of the week?"

Miller's idea is illustrated in Figure 1.1, where the x-axis gives the amount of information received and the y-axis how much information is reproduced correctly. Take, for example, a test in which you are asked to repeat a string of numbers read out to you. The y-axis shows how many numbers you repeat correctly. If you hear two numbers, you can easily remember them and tap them into a keyboard. You are on the straight part of the graph, where information input is the same as output. But if you are asked to repeat twelve numbers, or twenty, you will probably be able to tap in only seven of them correctly. You are now on the part of the graph where the curve bends under the confines of your capacity. Your copper wires just can't take any more.

Half a century after Miller published his article, we find ourselves in something of an information renaissance. Computerization, which was still in its cradle in the early 1950s, has exploded into every nook and cranny of our societies, cultures, and lifestyles. Information technology is now starting to present us with such a surplus of information per unit of time that the capacity limitations of our brains, what Miller calls the "channel capacity," has become a very real matter for our daily lives.

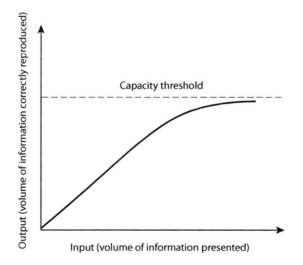

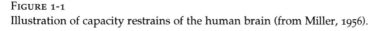

FIGURE 1-1
Illustration of capacity restrains of the human brain (from Miller, 1956).

■ The Stone Age Brain

If we have an inherent limitation to our ability to handle information, Miller's inbuilt mental bandwidth, it is probably hundreds of thousands of years old. Anatomically modern *Homo sapiens* evolved some 200,000 years ago in Africa. Geneticists have shown that every living human has DNA from one and the same woman, humanity's Eve, who lived at some point between 150,000 and 200,000 years ago. *Homo sapiens* then dispersed out into the world, including to southern Europe, where they gradually displaced their contemporaries the Neanderthals. Early people here left behind magnificent cave paintings, such as those in the cave of Cro-Magnon in southern France, which lent its name to this modern type of *Homo sapiens*.

Cro-Magnonshad the same brain volume and anatomy as we have today and if we were to dress one up in modern clothes, he would raise few eyebrows as he walked the streets of a modern city.

Cro-Magnon humans lived a leisurely life as hunters and gatherers, probably spending most of their days in groups of a few families, possibly fifty individuals. Occasionally the clan, a larger grouping of roughly 150 related individuals, would gather. Most of their time was probably devoted to collecting and preparing food, preparing skins, making tools, and going on the odd hunt. The technological environment in which Cro-Magnons lived consisted of a mere handful of tools, such as arrowheads, needles, and bone hooks.

The brains with which we are born today are almost identical to those with which Cro-Magnons were born forty thousand years ago. If there is some inherent limitation to our ability to handle information, it should be present already at this time, when the most technologically advanced artifact was the barbed bone harpoon. The same brain now has to take on the torrent of information that the digital society discharges over us. A Cro-Magnon human met in one year as many people as you and I can meet in one day. The volume and complexity of the information we're expected to handle continues to increase. If there are any inbuilt limitations that serve as some kind of shutoff valve, what mental functions are we then talking about? Where will we find the bottleneck in the brain's capacity to process information?

▓ Brain Plasticity

What complicates and enriches the discussion on the Cro-Magnon brain and Miller's mental bandwidth is the recent discoveries concerning brain plasticity. After you have read this book, you will never again be the person you were before. This is not because the contents of this book will have any revolutionary effect on how you live your life, but because all types of experience and learning modify the brain. You never, as the man said, step into the same river twice.

The brain doesn't change only as it stores memories. Different functions are located at different sites around the brain, so we can talk about a functional brain map. What scientists have found is that rather than being static, this map is forever being redrawn. Much of our knowledge of how the brain changes comes from studies of what happens when it is deprived of information input. When a person loses a limb and the corresponding part of the sensory cortex no longer receives information from those particular nerves, surrounding areas of the brain will start to fill the space. If you lose an index finger, the area of the brain that once received signals from that finger will shrink; the adjacent area, which receives signals from the middle finger, will expand. The brain map has been redrawn.

An even greater information deficit is the loss of visual information in the blind. Measurements of the brain activity of blind people when reading Braille show that the visual areas of their brains are activated despite the absence of any actual visual perceptions. It thus seems as if the people are using their visual cortex to process other sensory information instead. We could therefore be looking at the same plasticity as when the brain receives no sensory information from a lost finger: surrounding areas expand and take over the unused part of the brain. Similar results have been obtained from studies of people who were born deaf, in which scientists have seen activity in the auditory areas when their subjects read sign language.

The brain changes not only when we lose information but also when we are exposed to excessive activation—for example, when we practice a skill, such as learning a musical instrument, with year-in, year-out, hour-after-hour drills. When scientists mapped the areas that receive sensory information from the left hand of string musicians, they found that the area activated by sensory impressions is larger than that in nonplayers. They also found that the area of the brain activated on hearing piano notes is roughly 25 percent larger in pianists than in nonmusicians, and that the pathways conducting motor impulses differ.

Juggling is not something that many people do on a daily basis. But if we were to start practicing, we'd improve markedly in just a few weeks. It is, in other words, an activity that lends itself to the study of what happens in the brain when a specific activity is learned. One study examined the structure of the brain in a group of subjects before and after a three-month course in juggling. What the scientists found was that an area in the occipital lobe specializing in the perception of motion grew over this period, but three months after training stopped it had shrunk again, and lost roughly half the increase previously induced by training. In other words, as little as three months' activity, or three months' passivity, had an immediate effect on brain structure.

What still remains something of a puzzle is how the constant mental demands of the information society influence our brains. Do they have a "training" effect on the brain, just as other types of exercise and learning do?

■ Increases in IQ During the Twentieth Century

When, in the 1980s, the New Zealand sociologist James Flynn was carrying out what he thought would be a routine check of historical IQ test scores, he discovered something that would cause a stir in the world of psychology for decades to come: it seemed as if people's IQs were increasing. This phenomenon is known today as the Flynn effect.

By definition, the average IQ score of the entire population is 100. After a new version of an IQ test is administered to a large cohort of people—eighteen-year-olds, for example—it is adjusted to give an average result of 100. During such tests, subjects are often asked to take the old IQ test as well to see if performances on both tests agree. What Flynn discovered was that each time a group of people was tested, they performed better on the old test. When a group of eighteen-year-olds took a twenty-year-old test, they no longer scored 100 like their coevals of twenty years before, but always slightly higher. Flynn looked at more than seventy studies including a total of more than 7,500 participants between 1932 and 1978 and found that the average IQ increased by 3 points, roughly 3 percent, per decade.

What is so sensational about these findings is the degree of increment. In sixty years—that's two generations—scores have risen by roughly one standard deviation. This means that an eighteen-year-old who scored the average for his cohort in 1990 would, if transported sixty years back in time, be among the highest-performing sixth. From being

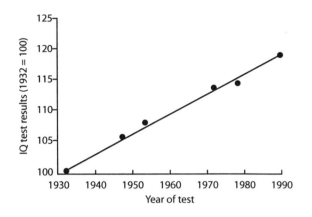

FIGURE 1-2
Changes in IQ during the 1900s (from Flynn, 1987).

an average student in a class of thirty, he would suddenly find himself in the top five.

Obviously this rise in IQ scores could be put down to educational improvements; however, if this were so, we would expect the greatest gains in tests measuring vocabulary and general knowledge, with lower gains on tests of problem-solving activities, which are generally considered culture-neutral and relatively impervious to level of education. However, when he looked in closer detail at the changes in the American IQ tests, he found that the exact opposite was the case: the increase was more marked for problem-solving activities, while there was hardly any change at all for the tests measuring vocabulary.

To verify this, Flynn made an international comparison of the results of problem-solving activities called Raven's matrices (which are specifically designed to reflect fluid intelligence, regardless of acquired knowledge; see page 42). After analyzing the trends over time in the results recorded by almost everyone who'd been tested on entering the military from 1952 to 1982 in Israel, Norway, Belgium, Holland,

and England, Flynn noted the same effects that had previously been observed in the American IQ tests, with the gains being made at almost exactly the same rate across the countries. When problem-solving abilities were analyzed in isolation, the increase was even greater, nearly twice what had been observed in average scores on tests comprising both verbal and problem-solving tasks.

Increases in IQ scores are corroborated by an overwhelming volume of data from different studies and are considered indubitable. On the other hand, no one can say with any certainty to what the effect is attributable. James Flynn himself first thought that these figures could not correspond to an improvement in intelligence "for real." The case of the eighteen-year-old who would be a star student if transported sixty years back in time just didn't add up, he argued. Instead, Flynn used the phenomenon of rising test results to denounce the use of the tests in the first place. Unfortunately, he didn't really have any argument for this other than it seeming counterintuitive for people to have become generally more intelligent. Flynn's interpretation that IQ tests are unreliable also failed to win much support among his fellow psychologists. Now, most psychologists—including Flynn, who seems to have changed tack himself—believe that the increase in test scores reflects a genuine improvement in people's ability to solve problems "for real."

No single factor has been identified that can explain the Flynn effect. One fascinating possibility is that it is factors in our mental environments that account for much of the change. Could it be the case that the greater flow of information has a training effect and that ever-increasing mental demands are helping to boost people's intelligence? If so, exactly which of the mental demands around us give rise to this improvement? Which functions can be practiced, and under what circumstances?

■ The Future

Our understanding of the human brain has grown exponentially in the past few decades. Now, for the first time, researchers are able to make links between limitations in information processing and cerebral function. Brain research has little to contribute to Miller's rhetorical question about the seven daughters of Atlas or the seven wonders of the world. But in the search for the factors that define the bottleneck in the brain's limitations, scientists have started to round up a few prime suspects. This book is about how they have gone about hunting them out.

If we learn more about our mental limitations and where they are located in the brain, we might also be able to understand how to change these functions through exercise or otherwise. In 2004, a number of well-known neuroscientists, including Nobel laureate Eric Kandel, wrote a review of these new possibilities and of the ethical dilemmas they raise. The article begins: "Humanity's ability to alter its own brain function might well shape history as powerfully as the development of metallurgy in the Iron Age." The review was entitled "Neurocognitive Enhancement: What Can We Do and What Should We Do?" This is a question that concerns every one of us.

I will be describing a little of what the latest brain research tells us about our attentional abilities, information processing, and brain training. This is not a textbook that aims to cover all the research being conducted on memory and attention. Even if I had the capacity to embrace such a large area (which I don't), there'd be few readers with the time to plow through such an epic—too much information, too little time. Instead, I have tried to write a book on a series of associated studies that together build up a story. I will be drawing on as many bits of information as we need to piece together a jigsaw puzzle that gives at least part of the picture, even if it doesn't reproduce the entire scene.

This story will also include my own research into brain function, which concerns, among other points of inquiry, limitations on simultaneous performance and how mental abilities can be actively developed.

There is general concern about what the fast pace of society is doing to our mental well-being. Books and magazines are full of advice on how we can learn to be less stressed, lower the demands on ourselves, and take life easier: slow cities, slow food, time for reflection, and so forth. It all has its place. But this book sends an opposing and more optimistic message. It proposes that we must also acknowledge our thirst for information, stimulation, and mental challenges. It is arguably when we determine our limits and find an optimal balance between cognitive demand and ability that we not only achieve deep satisfaction but also develop our brain's capacity the most.

But before we reach that point in our story, let us first look more closely at the mental demands that surround us. What is attention? How do we keep information in the brain, and can this ability be manipulated?

2 ∎

The Information Portal

Let us return to Linda. There she is, sitting at her desk in her open-plan office, surrounded by chatting colleagues and ringing phones. Her desk is littered with reports, articles, and brochures. On her computer screen is a Web page displaying an inventory of hard disks from which she has to select one for purchase. To the right are small animated advertisements for bargain trips to the West Indies. A little icon along the bottom edge of the screen reminds her that she has not yet emptied her inbox, and her cell phone announces with a happy *pling* that she has just received a text message. What choice should she make? Where should she even direct her gaze, and what elements of her visual field should she take in, process, understand, and think about? Where should she direct her attention?

Attention is the portal through which the information flood reaches the brain. Directing your attention at something is analogous to selecting information, as you give priority to only a small part of all the information available.

Attention is often likened to a beam of light or a spotlight. In much the same way as you can aim a flashlight at a certain object in a darkened room, you can direct your attention at selected parts of your surroundings and choose a small amount of information from everything around you.

If we are to sort out what happens when the Cro-Magnon brain meets the information flood, we must start here, with attention.

■ Different Kinds of Attention

Linda finally decides to ignore her e-mails and begins reading one of the reports stacked up on her desk. Calm reigns for a little while, and she gets through a good many pages without too much difficulty. But she soon realizes that she has not understood a word of what she has read in the past minute, as she has been thinking about what happened during dinner the evening before.

When she becomes aware that her thoughts are drifting away, she makes herself refocus on the text. However, just a minute or so later she becomes distracted by someone dropping a coffee cup on the floor behind her, which attracts not only Linda's attention but that of the entire office. Early morning turns into late morning, and the general level of activity in the office is so high that Linda decides that she might as well leave the reports until later.

Later that afternoon, when the office has started to empty, Linda resumes her reading. She now manages to concentrate for a full forty-five minutes, with the help of a little caffeine, until the density of the prose and a little lack of sleep conspire to bring on an unshakable tiredness that compels her to put the ream of paper back onto her desk.

Obviously, Linda's problem with the day's report reading is related to attention. So what are our "attentional abilities"? Scientists researching cerebral function and attention have identified different kinds attention. There are at least three, for example, involved in Linda's attempts to do her work. The first is *controlled attention*, which she uses when she consciously forces herself to read the report. When her thoughts wandered to the dinner of the previous evening, she lost control of her attention. The second type is *stimulus-driven attention*, which is involuntarily attracted to an unexpected event in a person's immediate environment—such as the coffee cup hitting the ground. The third type is *arousal*, which became a problem later in the day as tiredness descended upon her.

This book will be concentrating on the first two types of attention, those concerned with selectivity. Before we proceed, however, let us look a little more closely at arousal. Arousal differs slightly from the other types of attention in that it does not select a specific point in the room or a specific object. It is, as we say, nonselective. Levels of arousal can vary from second to second and from hour to hour. The typical example used to illustrate arousal patterns is soldiers on radar duty, scanning their radar screens for hours on end for small dots representing potential enemy aircraft. During such tasks, which offer few stimuli, arousal slowly declines, a phenomenon that can be measured as poorer performances and slower reaction times.

Levels of arousal can be temporarily raised with a warning of some impending event. Certain substances, caffeine for one, can also help to give a short-term boost to arousal—two cups in the late evening will improve the performance of our radar operators. However, soldiers who drink ten cups of coffee will be less effective at their task, as they might very well interpret every new dot on the screen as an enemy aircraft. Everything in moderation, as they say. The relationship between arousal and performance follows a curve resembling an inverted U: we perform best at moderate levels of arousal, where performance reaches an optimum between the extremes of too little and too much (Figure 2.1). In some respects, stress can have the same effect on the brain as coffee. Moderate levels of stress can thus be beneficial; excessive levels of stress preclude optimal performance.

■ Absentmindedness

If we do not focus our attention on something, we will not remember it. Absentmindedness is one of the most common causes of forgetfulness—or, as memory researcher and author Daniel Schacter puts it, one of the "seven sins of memory." A dramatic illustration of this is the story of the missing Stradivarius. A string quartet has just performed a concert in Los Angeles, one of the violinists having played on a particularly valuable violin, a priceless seventeenth-century Stradivarius. After the concert, the quartet gets ready to drive back to their hotel. The violinist, no doubt tired after the performance and perhaps with his mind on how well they have played and the morning's reviews,

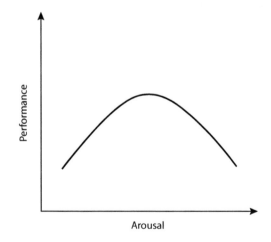

FIGURE 2-1
The relationship between arousal and performance.

absentmindedly places the violin on the roof of the car as he climbs in. The car drives off, and when they arrive, he realizes that his violin is missing—a mystery that remains unresolved for twenty-seven years until it is identified in a workshop, where it has been handed in for repair. This demonstrates how attention is essential, albeit insufficient at times, to our ability to store information in our memories. If your attention is directed elsewhere when you put your glasses down, it will be difficult for you to remember later where you left them. The information never made it through the portal.

When we direct our attention toward a place or an object, we become better and more efficient at interpreting its information content and are more able to detect slight changes in its appearance. If Linda is on her way home late at night and thinks she spies someone lurking in a doorway, she will stop and focus all her attention on that spot. She will not ignore another figure appearing in a neighboring doorway, but she will be better at detecting subtle shifts in the shadows surrounding the doorway on which she has focused her attention. Her attention will not only improve her ability to perceive changes but also speed up her reaction time should a menacing silhouette emerge from out of the gloom.

■ Measuring Attention in Milliseconds

We all have a subjective feeling of what attention is. Scientists, however, feed on precision and like to measure whatever it is they happen to be studying. And attention actually can be quantified.

Psychologist Michael I. Posner at the University of Oregon is the creator of a series of simple yet ingenious experiments that can be carried out on a computer and that each require a different kind of attention. In one, the test subject is asked to press a button as soon as she sees a little square target appear on the screen. As this event occurs without warning, her task is mainly one of stimulus-driven attention. In another, a triangle appears to alert the subject to the appearance of the target. This increases her arousal. In a third, an arrow appears on the screen a few seconds before the target, telling the subject not only that the event will occur soon but also where. The subject can now, by controlling her attention, direct her attentional spotlight onto a particular location on the screen in anticipation of the target's appearance.

By measuring reaction times during such tests, scientists have been able to quantify different kinds of attention; interestingly, what they find is that they seem fairly independent of one another. Such systemic autonomy also means that we can have problems with one kind of attention without this necessarily affecting the others.

This phenomenon was picked up by an Australian study in which children with and without diagnosed ADHD were asked to play two different games on a Sony PlayStation. The first was Point Blank, which involves aiming at and shooting various targets. The children had to respond as quickly as they could by pressing a button, their success rates being determined largely by their stimulus-driven attention. The second game was Crash Bandicoot, a platform game in which players have to navigate the brave little bandicoot (a kind of marsupial rat) along a preset path through the jungle while performing tasks, avoiding traps, and achieving certain goals. Unlike the first game, in which the subjects simply have their attention grabbed by some moving object on the screen to which they have to react, the second requires a certain amount of attention control as well. The study found no performance disparity between the two groups when playing Point Blank; when playing Crash Bandicoot, however, the children with ADHD significantly underperformed those of the control group, scoring fewer points and causing the dynamic little bandicoot to die more often.

So it seems as if the two systems for stimulus-driven and controlled attention are somehow separated. By extension, this could mean that there are different parts of the brain, or different brain processes, controlling them. What, then, are the biological mechanisms behind attention? How is an attention spotlight encoded by our brain cells?

■ The Spotlight in the Brain

Imagine that you are standing in a large white room, very much like a medical examination room. Around the walls are boxes full of disposable gloves, surgical tape, and compresses; there is also a set of different-sized white and blue plastic balls and objects that look like enormous helmets fitted with protective grilles. The objects piled up against the walls have one thing in common: they are not magnetic. For in the middle of the room is a white cube about six feet on a side, containing an electromagnet with the capacity to generate a magnetic field powerful enough to make a lethal projectile of a nearby oxygen cylinder. To create such a powerful field, the superconductive coils must be cooled with liquid helium to a temperature of -269°C. In the middle of the cube is a cylindrical hole through which a horizontal bench can be slid, transporting anyone lying on it into the middle of the magnet to have her brain activity scanned.

The cube is a magnetic resonance (MR) scanner, one of the most sophisticated tools available if we want to look inside the brain to see how attention works. Once the subject is placed inside the scanner, she can be asked to perform certain mental tasks, such as shifting her attention from one part of a picture to another, while the MR scanner captures images of her brain. After about half an hour of this, enough information has been recorded to pinpoint which parts of the brain have been activated.

Essentially, the technique involves the analysis of the blood flow in the brain. When the nerve cells, or neurons, of a particular area are activated, the supply of oxygenated blood to them increases. In the 1990s, scientists discovered that since the presence or absence of an oxygen molecule in hemoglobin (a component of blood) affects the magnetic field, an MR scanner could be used to obtain images of brain activity. The MR scanner can also be used to create detailed pictures of brain anatomy in order to locate tumors and other anomalies. However, when the MR scanner is used in a way that makes it sensitive to changes in oxygenated hemoglobin, it is brain function that scientists are interested in. The technique is therefore called functional magnetic resonance imaging, or fMRI.

In one study, carried out by Julie Brefczynski and Edgar DeYoe at the Medical College of Wisconsin, fMRI was used to measure the effects of attention. The subjects were asked to lie inside the MR scanner and look at a screen displaying a circle divided into colored sectors like those of a dartboard. They were asked to keep their eyes fixed on the center point but to shift their attention from sector to sector. This was therefore a test of controlled attention. To make sure that brain activity was not affected by eye movement, they used the phenomenon of being able to separate where the eyes are focused and where the attention is directed. You can try this for yourself by fixing your gaze at the center of a clock face and letting your attention travel around the numbers.

To understand the results, we need a little more background about how sensory impressions are processed by the brain. When using an MR scanner to study cerebral function, scientists are often interested in the activity of the cortex. The cortex is the thin layer of gray matter encasing the rest of the brain (or cerebrum). Thanks to its familiar folds and grooves, the cortex has exceptionally high surface area in relation to the limited volume available in the cranium. The first area of the cortex that is activated by visual stimuli is the occipital lobe, also known as the primary visual cortex. From here, signals are sent to other, more specialized visual areas. Each part of a person's immediate surroundings, such as the sectors of the dartboard, is decoded by a different cortical visual area, making each one a kind of internal map of the outside world.

When the subjects kept their eyes still but moved their attention around the sectors, the scientists were able to detect activity in the corresponding parts of the primary visual cortex. In fact, the results were so clear that it was possible for them to determine where the subjects had directed their attention just by looking at where their brains were being activated. This study demonstrates that the analogy of a spotlight holds fast even when we are describing the biological mechanism of attention. If the visual area is a map of the surroundings, attention can be likened to a beam of light that illuminates specific parts of this map. If an area is thus illuminated, it means that there is a higher degree of activity in the neurons there, which makes them more receptive to information.

There are similar brain maps for the other senses. The somatosensory cortex of the brain, for instance, contains an anatomical map. In one of the first studies of brain activity and attention, neurophysiologist Per Roland asked subjects to shut their eyes and count how many times their index finger was stroked with a hair while he measured their brain activity. However, the instruction to the subjects was a bogus one, and the event never actually happened. Nevertheless, the simple fact that the subjects were expecting some sensation and therefore directing their attention toward their finger excited activity in the corresponding sensory area of the brain.

■ Competition Between Neurons

One study elegantly demonstrates how attention works by choosing, even down at the cellular level. Here, the researchers first registered the activity of a visual area in the brain when a monkey was shown a green circle either by itself or accompanied by a red circle. What they found was that the activity stimulated in the visual area when only the green circle was shown dropped when the two circles were shown together. Although this is probably attributable to the mutually suppressive effect of the neurons in two adjacent parts of the visual cortex, what is interesting was that when the monkey ignored the red circle and focused its attention on the green one, there was just as much brain activity as when the green circle was displayed on its own.

This experiment reveals one of the most rudimentary mechanisms of attention: the selection of neurons to be stimulated at the expense of others. The phenomenon is called *biased competition*. When there is just one object, in this case the single green circle, there is no need for attention; it is the amount of competing information to which our brains are exposed that impels a choice.

Can we now apply this knowledge to the situation at the office? If Linda has an office more resembling a monastery cell—austere and with only one text (a Bible?) on her desk—there is little demand on her attention and no need for her to make choices. However, as soon as she has two documents in front of her, she is forced to choose and direct her attention, and as the volume of information increases, these demands on her attention become even greater.

An interesting yet elusive aspect of attention that is how our thoughts, ideas, memories, and impulses compete for our attention with each other and with stimuli in our surroundings. If we have only one thought in our head, we are under no real pressure to control our attention. This pressure increases when we add impulses, memories, and thoughts. Interesting ideas and attractive impulses should attract attention in much the same way as external events automatically draw attention to themselves, such as when the person behind us drops a coffee cup on the floor or a bird suddenly flies into the room.

■ Two Parallel Systems of Attention

If the increased activity of the visual cortex—the illuminated map—is a final effect, what are the causes or sources of attention? Where is the spotlight? If we could measure brain activity at the moment an instruction to direct the attention toward a particular object is received, we should be able to locate the parts of the brain that exercise the control.

Several research groups have done just this experiment, using versions of Posner's tests of controlled attention. The results concur in identifying two areas, one in the parietal lobe and one in the superior part of the frontal lobe, that are active when we direct our attention. This could be the source of the brain's "light beam." Disregarding the other structures in the brain that are also involved, what may be happening is that neurons in these areas are contacting others in the visual areas and activating exactly the corresponding points on the map.

Scientists have also identified the areas that are activated on stimulus-driven attention (for example, when a target appears on a computer screen without advance warning). These different areas lie on the border between the parietal lobe and the temporal lobe and a little further down the frontal lobe. Figure 2.3 is a reproduction of the findings of Maurizio Corbetta and Gordon Shulman from Washington University, who compiled activation patterns of a variety of studies. Here, neuronal activity during controlled attention and stimulus-driven attention is delineated with a white ring and a black ring, respectively. It seems, therefore, that there are two parallel systems for attention, one for controlled attention and one for stimulus-driven attention, thus corroborating the psychological experiments demonstrating that the two different types of attention are mutually independent.

Absentmindedness, as in the story of the violin on the car roof, is a form of attention breakdown that all of us

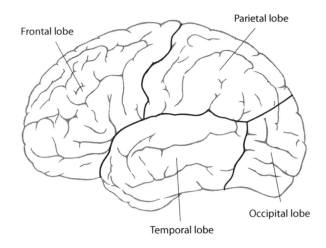

FIGURE 2-2
The lobes of the brain.

suffer to one extent or another. However, there are people with serious attention impairment, particularly with respect to the systems for stimulus-driven attention. The phenomenon is termed *neglect* and is caused by damage around the parietal lobe. The area of the parietal lobe in the

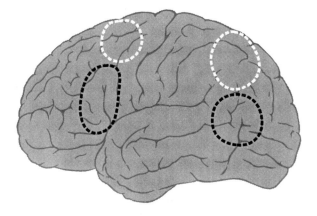

FIGURE 2-3
Areas responsible for stimulus-driven attention (black circles) and controlled attention (white circles). Adapted from Corbetta and Shulman (2002).

left cerebral hemisphere processes information from the right-hand visual field, while that of the right hemisphere processes information from both parts of the visual field. On injury to the left hemisphere, therefore, the right can function as a backup system; the right, however, cannot count on such a reciprocal service, and the symptoms of the lesion become more salient. People with this kind of injury start to "neglect" one-half of their visual field; if someone with neglect is asked to draw a picture of a clock, he or she completes only one-half of the face.

In one study, a woman with a lesion in her parietal lobe was asked to shut her eyes and describe a familiar public square in her Italian hometown. She was asked to imagine that she was standing at one end of this square facing the church, and to describe the different buildings around her. Because of her injury, however, she could describe only those in her right visual field. She was then asked to imagine walking up to the church and turning to regard the square from the opposite direction. Doing this, she was able to describe the buildings on the other side.

Certain limitations in the brain's ability to receive information can thus be attributed to the mechanisms of attention. However, if we want to explain the limitations on more complex mental activities, the really interesting constraints lie in how we can control our attention and how we retain the information we absorb. So how does this happen?

3 ∎
The Mental Workbench

Sometimes our attention can be drawn automatically to certain changes in our surroundings. As for controlled attention, however, some kind of instruction is needed for where it is to be directed. If our intention is to direct and fix our attention onto a predetermined target, let us say a face in a crowd, we have to have some sort of memory of this target while we are searching for it. How do we remember what it is we are to concentrate on?

∎ Working Memory

The answer is *working memory*. The term refers to our ability to remember information for a limited period of time, usually a matter of seconds. To all appearance it might seem a simple function, but it is fundamental and vital to numerous mental tasks, from attention control to solving logical problems. As working memory will run like a thread through the rest of the book, we will dedicate this chapter to the concept of working memory and how it relates to other functions.

Let us return again to Linda in her hectic office environment. When, for example, she is busy searching for a stamp in that cluttered top desk drawer of hers, she has to keep in her working memory what she is looking for. The untidiness of her desk presents a myriad of different objects that compete for her attention. The neurons in the visual areas of her brain compete for which are to be activated, and so she needs to control her attention. Maybe she becomes so distracted by the mess that she shuts the drawer and starts doing something else only to ask herself two seconds later why she just shut that drawer or where the stamp is. The instruction to herself to look for the stamp has vanished from her working memory.

You use your working memory when directory assistance gives you a number that you have to remember until you have found a piece of paper and a pen that works. In this case, what you are trying to keep in your working memory is verbal information, usually by repeating the numbers quietly to yourself. Chess is an example of when we hold visual information in working memory: "If I move my knight there, he'll take it with his bishop, but then I'll take his bishop with my queen." Here we are running a kind of visual simulation in our heads and need working memory to remember all the simulated moves.

Although the term "working memory" was already being used back in the 1960s by neuroscientist Karl Pribram, Alan Baddeley is the psychologist who is most often credited with having defined it, in its most common usage, in the early 1970s. He posited three components to working memory: one responsible for storing visual information, termed the *visuospatial sketch pad;* one responsible for storing verbal information, termed the *phonological loop;* and one central component coordinating the other two, termed the *central executive.* Allan Baddeley has also proposed another kind of working memory store, the *episodic buffer*, which retains episodic information in working memory. This buffer is, however, less well characterized than the other components. When remembering chess moves, you are using the visuospatial sketch pad; when remembering a telephone number, it is the phonological loop that comes in handy. Both cases need some kind of coordination, and this is where the central executive comes in.

If a psychologist wants to test your verbal working memory, she might ask you to repeat a series of numbers. If she wants to test your visuospatial working memory, she may use a test called "block repetition," in which you will have to remember the order in which the tester points at different blocks. First she tries two blocks. This test passed, she will advance you to a new sequence of three blocks, and so forth. When you have reached perhaps seven blocks you will probably start making mistakes, and when you have reached a level where you have only a 50 percent chance of remembering the entire sequence correctly (i.e., when you make a mistake roughly every other time), you have reached the limits of your working memory capacity. This is a measure of the amount of information you can retain in your working memory.

One of the defining characteristics of working memory is this very limitation. This is what was illustrated in the introduction with the example of the directions: if you are told "Go straight ahead for two blocks and then left one block," you will have no difficulty remembering where to go. However, when the instruction is so prolix that it exceeds the capacity of your working memory, you could well find yourself lost.

■ Long-Term Memory

The capacity limitation of working memory is one of the things that distinguishes it from long-term memory.

In long-term memory, we memorize events in which we have been involved, such as what we ate for dinner yesterday. We can also remember facts unassociated with a specific learning occasion, such as the meaning of a word or the capital of Morocco. Our memory for events is called *episodic memory*, the one for facts *semantic memory*. The amount of information that can be stored in the long-term memory is virtually boundless. Long-term memory means that we can memorize something, direct our attention at something else for a few minutes or years, and then retrieve the first item again at will. This is not how working memory operates, for when information is being stored here, it is under the constant glare of attention.

Memories are encoded into long-term storage through a chain of biochemical and cellular processes. Brain areas that are important for the memory at an early stage, such as the hippocampus in the temporal lobe, are less so later on. A dramatic illustration of this is the effect of electroconvulsive therapy as a treatment for depression. After such a shock, long-term memories in an early and more unstable phase of encoding can become disturbed, rendering patients unable to remember things they had experienced a few days or even weeks ago while retaining memories that were encoded a year before.

Let us take an everyday example of the difference between long-term memory and working memory. If you park your car outside a supermarket in order to buy a quart of milk, it is your long-term memory you use to remember where your car is. Your parking spot is nothing you continuously visualize as you walk around the shop, but information that you encode for subsequent retrieval. Your working memory, on the other hand, you might use to remember, as you lose yourself among the aisles, that it is a quart of milk you have gone in to buy.

So working memory is normally used to keep information active for a few seconds, while long-term memory can

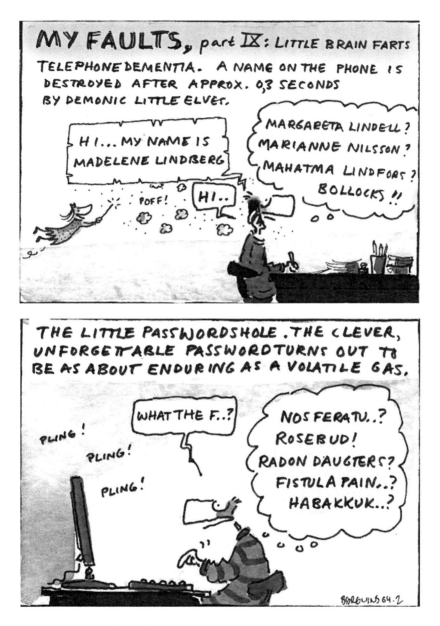

FIGURE 3-1 AND FIGURE 3-2
Cartoonist Berglin captures perfectly the differences between working memory and long-term memory with his illustration of a working memory problem (telephone dementia) and a long-term memory problem (the little password hole). © Jan Berglin.

keep it stored for years on end. However, the difference between the two is found in how the brain stores the information, not necessarily in exactly how long ago it was that you saw the thing you later remember. One evening a friend of mine met a nice young woman in a bar. When they parted she gave him her phone number. The problem was that he had nothing on which to write it down, and he did not dare rely on his long-term memory. Instead, he kept the number in his working memory by silently repeating it to himself on his way home while carefully avoiding looking at car license plates, bus numbers, and other such distracting groups of digits. Once home, twenty minutes later, he finally got to scribble the number down on a scrap of paper. They are now happily married with two children.

■ Controlling Attention

In the 1970s, neurophysiologists began studying working memory in primates, particularly macaques. A macaque weighs in at about twenty-two pounds, and its brain is a mere two inches long. Macaques are not that intelligent, not even compared with chimpanzees, but they can retain information in their working memories, which have a capacity thought to be roughly equivalent to that of a one-year-old human.

Exceedingly simple tasks were therefore needed for the monkeys to perform. One early test involved hiding a peanut under one of two cups while the monkey was watching, concealing the cups from the monkey with a curtain, and then drawing the curtain to reveal the cups and let the monkey make its choice. If the monkey retained information in its working memory about where the peanut had been hidden, it would choose the correct cup. However, it was impossible to rule out the possibility that the monkey oriented its body toward the cup with the peanut, stared at the place where it was hidden, or used other little ruses to solve the problem. To cancel out the effect of eye movements, scientists devised something called the *oculomotor delay response task*, but for simplicity's sake we will just call it the "dot test."

For the dot test, the monkey is trained to fix its gaze onto an image of a cross directly in front of it. A dot is then flashed on the periphery of the screen. After a delay of a few seconds, the cross disappears, upon which the monkey has to shift its gaze onto the position where it registered the dot. During this time, therefore, the monkey has to keep this location in its working memory.

Remembering the position of dots and then transferring our gaze there is not how most of us would feel we use our working memories in our daily lives. The dot test is, in fact, so unnatural that performing it takes weeks for monkeys to learn. However, it is ingenious in that it isolates the essence of working memory: making a response not based on what we see but on information retained in our heads. Much of what we know about how working memory is encoded in the brain derives from decades of studies using variations on this test.

If we look carefully at what is going on in the dot test, we find striking similarities with what happens in Posner's attention tests (see Figure 3.3). In one of his experiments, an arrow was used to indicate where the subject could expect the target to appear. The subject then had to keep her attention directed at that particular point. This test cannot be performed without the subject retaining positional information in her working memory, in exactly the same way as the monkeys have to remember the location of the dot. This demonstrates, in its very simplest form, the overlap between the control of attention on the one hand and working memory on the other. Working memory is essential for controlling attention. We have to remember what it is we are to concentrate on.

Posner's controlled attention test

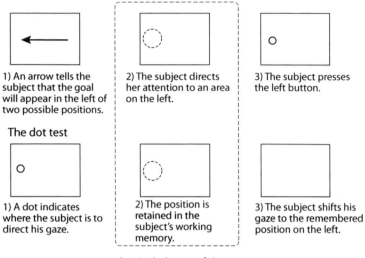

1) An arrow tells the subject that the goal will appear in the left of two possible positions.

2) The subject directs her attention to an area on the left.

3) The subject presses the left button.

The dot test

1) A dot indicates where the subject is to direct his gaze.

2) The position is retained in the subject's working memory.

3) The subject shifts his gaze to the remembered position on the left.

Identical phases of the two tests.

FIGURE 3-3
Similarities between a task measuring controlled attention and a working memory task (dot test).

Neurophysiologist Robert Desimone was one of the first scientists to make this connection explicit. He called the mnemonic component of the attention tests the *attentional template*, which is no more complicated than understanding that when we are scanning a crowd for a familiar face we have to retain in our working memory the target of our search. However, note also that the overlap between working memory and attention applies only to controlled attention; stimulus-driven attention requires no working memory.

■ Problem Solving

What makes working memory particularly interesting is that it not only retains instructions, numbers, and positions in the memory but also seems to play a critical part in our ability to solve problems. Te get a feel for this, do the following test: read the question in the next sentence once, shut the book, and work out your answer. What is 93—7 + 3?

How did you do? Now try to identify the mental operations that took place before you arrived at the solution. If you went about it like most people, you started by subtracting 7 from 93 to get 86. You then stored the information while consulting your memory about the next task, namely, to add 3. You then added 3 to 86. Operations such as this are impossible unless you can somehow remember both the question and the result of the intermediary mental acts you perform to arrive at the answer. Working memory is thus used like a workbench for performing different mental tasks.

Similarly, working memory is used to keep in our minds the component parts of a logical problem, such as this: "If it rains, the lawn gets wet. If the lawn is now wet, can we conclude that it has rained?" Solving such syllogisms, like performing mental arithmetic, requires us to manipulate information stored in working memory. Alan Baddeley therefore defines working memory thus: "The term working memory refers to a brain system that provides temporary storage and manipulation of the information necessary for such complex cognitive tasks as language comprehension, learning, and reasoning."

Figure 3.4 shows a type of problem-solving task often used by psychologists to assess general intellectual abilities. It has been used for many decades, exists in many different versions, and goes under the name "Raven's matrices." The task uses a three-by-three matrix of symbols, the bottom rightmost of which is missing. The subject is to work out the rules that dictate how the symbols change from one row to the next and one column to the next. Once she has deduced the pattern, she will be able to draw a conclusion about what missing symbol looks like and select it from a group of possible solutions.

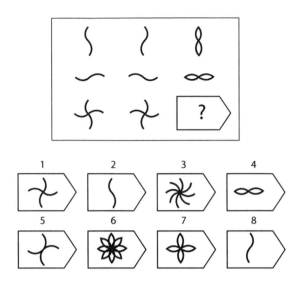

Figure 3-4
Raven's Matrices.

It turns out that our ability to solve such a problem depends significantly on how much information we are able to retain in working memory; in fact, one of the most-cited papers on this relationship is called "Reasoning Ability Is (Little More than) Working Memory Capacity?!" German psychologist Heinz-Martin Süß summarizes his results thus: "At present, working memory capacity is the best predictor for intelligence that has yet been derived from theories and research on human cognition."

Psychologist Randall Engle at the Georgia Institute of Technology in Atlanta has also shown that there is a strong correlation between the presentation of working memory tasks and problem-solving ability (or more exactly, gF—general fluid intelligence—which we will be discussing in the chapter on the Flynn effect). The relationship between working memory capacity and gF differs slightly depending on the test used, but a review paper reveals that the correlation usually lies between 0.6 and 0.8 (where 0 is no correlation and 1 is identity). This means that if we wish to explain why certain people are good at solving problems (such as Raven's matrices) and others not, roughly half of the difference, or half of the variance, can be attributed to differences in working memory capacity.

■ Working Memory Versus Short-Term Memory

The question often arises of what short-term memory is and how it relates to working memory. The answer is not that straightforward, and there is actually an ongoing academic debate on this issue. It has been noted that the ability to repeat a list of words that you have just heard has a very low correlation with gF, but performing a more complex verbal working memory task with dual-task requirements has a high correlation with gF. It has therefore been suggested that there are two classes of memory task, which many psychologists refer to as *short-term memory* and *working memory*. According to this dichotomy, short-term memory involves merely the retention and repetition of information, which has a low correlation with complex mental abilities and gF, while working memory denotes short-term memory tasks that require some kind of additional manipulation, contain some form of distraction, or demand a degree of simultaneous performance, and have a high correlation with gF.

The problem with this model of memory is that there is little consensus on which tasks are to be classified as what: some researchers would call repeating digits in reverse order a short-term memory task, while some call it a working memory task. It has also become clear that performance on short-term memory tasks with high information load is as highly correlated with gF as complex working memory tasks. Furthermore, the distinctions that apply to verbal working memory tasks do not seem to hold for visuo-spatial working memory tasks. Some visuospatial tasks without manipulation that require only retaining and repeating information are as correlated with gF as complex verbal working memory tasks. The definition that "working memory requires the retention and manipulation of information" thus does not hold up. As we shall discover in a later chapter, it also seems difficult to show any clear difference in brain activity between "short-term memory tasks" and "working memory tasks," at least within the visuo-spatial domain. It often appears to be the same brain area that is activated, although with varying intensity—which would suggest that what we are talking about is differences in degree rather than in kind.

Hopefully, we will one day have a nomenclature based on the brain activity observed during the performance of different working memory tasks. More about this later. At this point, it suffices to say that working memory tasks differ, but the term "working memory" will serve the purposes of this book. The main focus of our concern will henceforth be the visuospatial working memory, which is as highly correlated with gF as the complex verbal working memory tasks.

There are several reasons why working memory is so important to our problem-solving ability. To solve a Raven's matrix we need to retain and manipulate visual information in working memory while memorizing the instructions— just like in the little arithmetic problem above. Solving logical problems also seems to involve some kind of symbolic representation that is visuo-spatial in nature. But we also need to control our attention. In Randall Engle's interpretation, what is of particular importance is the overlap between working memory and the control of attention. We have to remember what it is we are to concentrate on.

4 ∎
Models of Working Memory

In chapter 3, we saw that the ability to retain information is essential to a wide range of mental tasks. Working memory is used to control attention, to remember instructions, to keep in mind a plan of things to do, and to solve complex problems. However, working memory is of limited capacity, a bottleneck that restricts our ability to process information and reason. If we were to ask ourselves what presents problems when the Stone Age brain meets the information flood, one of the answers would be the limitations of working memory. So let us now take a closer look at exactly how information is stored and whether we can localize where in the brain these limitations reside.

Some of the most important advances in our understanding of brain activity and working memory were made by Yale neuroscientist Patricia Goldman-Rakic, one of the developers of the dot test. When she was registering the activity of neurons in different parts of the primate brain, what she was looking for was activity clearly related to the various parts of the working memory experiment. This was quite a demanding search process, since most of the cells under observation did not seem to have anything to do with the tasks. For studies of this kind, an amplifier and speakers are connected to the sensors, reproducing the electrical activity of the neurons as a chaotic symphony of clicks and crackles—although chaotic it is not, of course; just too complex for us to understand.

However, out of this confusion Goldman-Rakic was able to extract certain patterns, the most interesting seeming to come from a number of cells activated during the period in which the information was being retained in working memory. These cells were active when the monkey looked at a dot it was to remember, and continued to send an uninterrupted current of signals even when the dot disappeared, right up to the point when the monkey shifted its gaze onto the memorized spot. This kind of activity was termed *delay-period activity*, and if it was interrupted, the monkey would no longer be able to remember the information. Nerve cells evincing this type of continual activity were found in the frontal lobes but alsoin the parietal lobes.

The theory advanced by Goldman-Rakic and others, such as Joaquin Fuster at the University of California, Los Angeles, is that the information is retained in working memory because certain neurons are continually active. This is a principle that differs from the way in which information is encoded in long-term memory, whereby interneuronal connections are permanently reinforced—a process that takes a long time and requires, among other things, the production of new proteins. The encoding of information in working memory is a much more dynamic process that provides an immediate means of storing information, since patterns of electrical activity can be established in a matter of milliseconds. However, it is also a sensitive means, since the memory will be lost once the network is disrupted and the continual surge of activity terminated.

We can refer back at this juncture to the question of how different kinds of memory are to be defined. If we want a nomenclature for mental functions to coincide with what happens in the brain, we could define working memory as the ability to keep information active for a short period, based on continual neuronal activity.

Let us now return to our example of parking the car in order to buy a quart of milk. The location of your car is stored in your long-term memory. No neurons in the frontal lobe are encoding its location or are continually active with this information as you browse the shelves. However, as you do so, the item for which you are searching—the milk—is stored in working memory. The information is "online," so to speak, in that it is constantly in your consciousness in a way that corresponds to the uninterrupted activity of certain frontal lobe neurons.

Just how the neurons manage to remain active during this delay period is still something of a mystery. One hypothesis is the presence of recurrent loops, neuronal networks that keep the activity going by stimulating each other. Research into these mechanisms has made some progress in recent years with the help of computer simulations. Built into these experiments are computer models of how individual neurons are activated; the virtual nerve cells are then linked together into networks, allowing scientists to examine the conditions under which the activity is maintained. It turns out that a delicate balance is needed between stimulation and inhibition. Too much inhibition, and the neuronal activity, and with it the information, dies out; too little inhibition, and the neuronal activity runs amok in a kind of virtual epilepsy.

■ The Information in the Parietal Lobe

Knowledge of how the human working memory operates started to pick up in the 1990s, when the development of

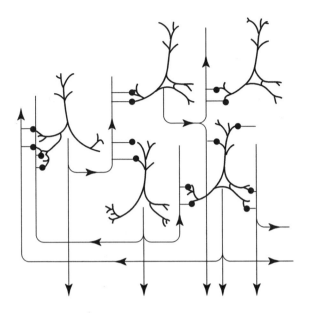

FIGURE 4-1
Computer models are used to explain how neuronal activity, and therefore information, can be retained by the coactivation of neuronal networks.

positron emission tomography (PET) made it possible for scientists to measure the cerebral blood flow of subjects performing working memory tasks. This revealed how the frontal lobe was activated, and correlated with previous knowledge of primate frontal lobe functionality and studies of frontal lobe lesions in humans. However, the PET scanner gives more detailed information, allowing researchers to distinguish areas that retain visual information from those active when retaining verbal information.

The PET scanner has a temporal resolution of only about a minute. In the mid-1990s, researchers started to use fMRI to take a snapshot of brain activity roughly every other second. With this higher temporal resolution, it is possible to delineate the activity generated by the presentation of an object during two distinct periods: the delay period, while the information is being retained in working memory, and the response. Several studies have analyzed the activity coincident with the delay period and have noted the persistent activity of the frontal lobes. The hypothesis that the information is retained by continual activity therefore seems to hold for humans. Naturally, the studies have given much more detailed results, such as the observation that it is not only the cortex of the frontal lobe that is continually active during the delay period but areas of the parietal lobe as well.

■ Memory and Attention Unified

By comparing the details from tests of controlled attention and tests of working memory, we would be able to see how working memory and the control of attention are linked, at least according to some psychological theories. But is it the same brain system that is being activated?

In one of the more ambitious studies of brain activity during working memory tasks, Clayton Curtis and Mark D'Esposito at the University of California, Berkeley, used the very same dot test procedures as had previously been used with monkeys. Fifteen people took part in the study, each having his or her brain activity measured for forty-five minutes while the researchers took snapshots of their brain activity at one-second intervals. This was a trial of endurance not only for the subjects, who had to lie inside an MR scanner for forty-five minutes remembering dots, but also for the researchers, who subsequently had to compile information from the forty thousand or so images obtained.

After analyzing these images statistically, Curtis and D'Esposito were able to spot activity in the parietal lobe (around the intraparietal sulcus), the upper part of the frontal lobe (the superior frontal gyrus), and the more anterior part of this same lobe (middle frontal gyrus). What is interesting is that the first two areas are the very same as those active in the experiments on controlled attention, such as Posner's (see page 29). As we can see, then, the results of the brain research substantiate the psychological description of the overlap between working memory and controlled attention. This could mean that there is no difference between remembering the position of a dot and remembering where to target the attention in anticipation of a dot yet to appear.

It should be added that the correspondence of working memory and attention control is not total. In many working memory tasks, there is activation further forward in the frontal lobe that is not always observed during attention tasks. Exactly what function this activity has is unclear. There is still much unknown territory on our map of cerebral function, an ignorance that applies particularly to the prefrontal lobes. It is possible, however, that activity here provides top-down control, stabilizing or boosting, for example, the connection between the upper parts of the frontal lobe and the parietal lobe.

■ How the Information Is Encoded

A crucial question concerning this neuronal activity is how the cells can remain active during the delay period without external stimulation. Feedback within networks of nerve cells seems to be a possible answer. Another important question is what type of information is encoded by this continual activity. What does it signify?

A similar issue has already been discussed by researchers into long-term memory. One theory says that certain nerve cells account for specific memories. This "grandmother cell theory" maintains that we have one particular cell that is activated each time we see our grandmother and that allows us to remember her.

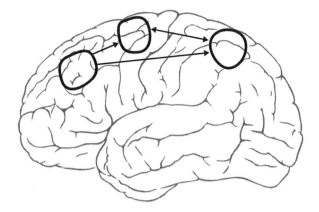

FIGURE 4-2

The ringed areas are those active during working memory tasks. An area of the parietal lobe and the upper part of the frontal lobe are continually active during the delay period of working memory tasks, when subjects are required to retain spatial information. These areas are identical to those activated on the control of attention. An area that is activated during working memory tasks but not always during controlled-attention tasks is located further forwards in the frontal lobe. The arrows indicate how the areas are thought to communicate with each other during working memory tasks (from Curtis and D'Esposito, 2003).

As regards working memory, one theory posits that the sensory information from the rear parts of the brain is conveyed to the specialized neurons of the frontal lobe in a way not dissimilar to the grandmother cell theory. Continual activity in a specific frontal lobe cell thus enables the monkey to remember that it saw a dot 90 degrees to the right; activity in a nearby cell corresponds to the memory of a dot 120 degrees to the right, and so forth. According to another model, information on different stimuli can be encoded by the particular frequency with which the neurons are activated. There are also studies, however, showing that the information cannot always be gleaned simply from the activity of the nerve cells in the frontal lobes. Certain cells exhibit working memory activity regardless of the type of stimulus being memorized. Since such a cell encodes for more than one sensory modality, such as phonic and visual information, we can call it *multimodal*—a kind of neuronal jack-of-all-trades.

All this may seem pedantic and academic, and without much relevance to anyone not exceptionally interested in cataloguing different kinds of nerve cell in the frontal lobes (which I admittedly am). However, how the information is encoded can have consequences for the manner in which the flow of information in the brain is organized. If each cell in the frontal lobe encodes for a specific stimulus, it suggests a parallel organization of the information flow. Goldman-Rakic, who advocated this model, argued that working memory comprises parallel systems, each of which processes its own kind of information. If, on the other hand, there are multimodal cells involved in working memory, they should receive information from sensory cells in the rear brain in what can be seen as a converging flow of information.

Some studies of working memory that my colleagues and I have performed are related to the debate on how information is encoded. In one experiment, brain activity was measured during two different working memory tasks, one involving memorizing tonal pitch and the other brightness. Certain areas in the brain were activated specifically during these working memory tasks, but independently of the kind of information being stored: multimodal working memory areas, in other words. This therefore confuted the parallel structure hypothesized by Goldman-Rakic, and has since been corroborated by other studies.

So what is the significance of these findings? The very fact that we have certain areas where information processing converges might well have a functional consequence. Parallel organization should be smoother, more free of disruption, and less capacity-restricting, in the same way as computers with parallel processors are superior to those with only one processor. Points of convergence are likely to form bottlenecks.

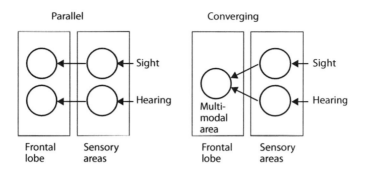

FIGURE 4-3
Illustration of the parallel and converging flow of information in the brain during working memory tasks.

If we are to look for a function that will present problems when the Stone Age brain meets the information flood, the limited capacity of working memory is a likely candidate. If we take a step further and seek the causes of the limitations of brain organization, the multimodal areas would seem to be possible bottlenecks. But what are we actually dealing with here? Can we find something as simple as individual areas in the brain that determine the capacity of our working memory or our ability to solve problems?

5 ■
The Brain and the Magical Number Seven

As mentioned above, George Miller established the hypothesis that there is a natural restriction on the human information-processing faculties that leaves us able to keep only roughly seven units in our working memory. One point of his was to transfer the bandwidth idea from information theory to psychology; in this sense the human brain could be seen as a channel of communication in which the volume of incoming information that can be stored, processed, and reproduced is fully quantifiable.

Comparing the brain to a copper wire is, of course, overly simplistic. Yet the questions remains: What is the cause of the brain's limited capacity to retain information in working memory? Can it be pinpointed to a specific brain area? What are the mechanisms that limit this capacity?

First, maybe we ought to point out that the number seven is not sacred. Just how much information working memory can hold is determined to a certain degree by how the tests are designed. If the information can be combined into meaningful units, such as KGB1968CIA2001, working memory is able to cope with more than seven items. Combing information into bits like this is called *chunking*. For other types of working memory task in which subjects are prevented from repeating the information to themselves during the delay period, the capacity of working memory drops to four units, as psychologist Nelson Cowan has shown. However, even though Cowan questions the specificity of the number seven, he agrees that there is a definite cutoff point, and that it is one of the most important limitations on the brain's capacity for processing information.

The fact also remains that if we ask twenty students to remember a series of random digits, most of them will be able to repeat between six and eight of them. If we test their visuospatial memories, some will remember five positions and some eight; whatever the results, the average will often lie remarkably close to Miller's limit of seven.

For a scientist, information is equivalent to variance, or differences. To assess, for instance, the effect of lead on cerebral development, we would have to examine the brains of people who had been exposed to a lot of lead, and compare them with the brains of people who had been exposed to little. So if we are to explore the relationship between brain capacity and function, we need to study differences in capacity. The most obvious differences in this respect are those between the working memories of children and adults, so let us take a little closer look at capacity development during childhood and at what happens in the brain as it is taking place.

■ The Maturing Brain

The next time you meet a seven-month-old baby, have a go at hiding her favorite toy under one of two blankets while the baby watches (having asked her parents' permission first, of course). Distract the baby's gaze for a few seconds and then let her try to find her toy. Repeat the experiment again and again, changing the hiding place each time to prevent the baby from using her long-term memory to remember where the toy is hidden.

A five-month-old baby is unable to perform this task successfully, as she is unable to retain a representation of an object she no longer sees: out of sight, out of mind. If you want to try to imagine what a life without a working memory would be like (and if imagining yourself as a goldfish is far too alien to you), try to see the world through the eyes of a baby: as a continual influx of impressions. At some time around the age of seven months, working memory slowly starts to develop, so by the age of about twelve months the baby is able to locate her hidden toy with a delay period of several seconds.

Remembering where the toy is hidden is the first little step on the road to working memory development. However, working memory continues to improve its capacity for storing information throughout childhood and into adolescence, which means that adults have a better working memory than children. When an eight-year-old is asked by his teacher to "take out your pencil, eraser, math book, and paper, turn to page twenty-five, and start doing the problems," the chances of him sitting there a minute later with his math book turned to the right page are rather small. It *could* be because he wants to continue playing, but it could also be due to the fact that his working memory has been overloaded, rendering him unable to retain the long string of instructions in his working memory all the way to successful completion.

There are many components to this development. One is the construction of strategies. A four-year-old, for instance, will not use silent repetition to remember numbers—a strategy that first appears at the age of six or seven. However, even if we ignore differences in strategy, a difference in working memory remains. This can be measured using simple tests in which children are asked to remember the position of dots shown to them one at a time. Several studies have demonstrated how a person's capacity to do this increases through childhood and early adulthood, reaching a plateau at around the age of twenty-five. For an eight-year-old, this development gives an increment in information storage of roughly 7 percent a year. Psychologists Sandra Hale and Astrid Fry have shown that this determines how our problem-solving ability improves during childhood. The bad news is that the capacity then enters a slow decline; according to some studies, we would be back at the level of a twelve-year-old by the age of fifty-five. Perhaps we oldies who have crossed the twenty-five-year threshold can draw some consolation from our ability to compensate for this deterioration with our accumulated knowledge and strategies. Or as a Greek saying has it, "Old age and treachery will overcome youth and skill."

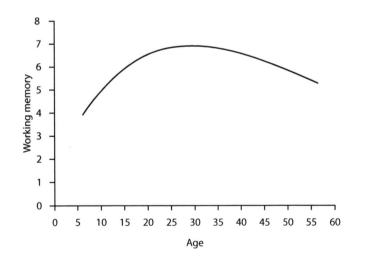

FIGURE 5-1
Changes in working memory during a person's life (from Swanson, 1999).

The claim that children have a worse working memory than adults does not seem to tally with the experiences that many parents (including myself) have of losing at Concentration to their children. Concentration (also known as Memory or Pairs), as most of you probably know, is a game made up of identical pairs of picture cards. Twenty or so such cards (i.e., ten or so pairs) are shuffled and laid out facedown. Players take turns flipping over two cards at a time; if the cards match, they are removed and added to the player's stack. The idea is for the players to remember the position of the different cards so that they can turn them over when needed. Systematic studies have been made of this game. As many have found to their chagrin, ten-year-olds, on average, beat their middle-aged parents, who can subsequently seek solace in trouncing their own elderly parents. This is because long-term memory comes in very handy in this game, as the information about the hidden faces of the cards is not something that we continually run over in our working memories, but rather is encoded into long-term memory for later retrieval. This use of long-term memory is exactly the same as when we remember where we parked the car after a brief shopping expedition. Some types of long-term memory skill are not subject to gradual development and can actually be better in children.

An electronic game called Simon is another kind of memory tester. One version has a circle of four different-colored buttons arranged in a circle that illuminate in a certain sequence, say, up-down-left-right. The point of the game is to press the buttons and repeat the sequence, which, if the player is successful, is then lengthened by one step: up-down-left-right-left. Many people claim to be able to remember a sequence of perhaps fifteen steps, which seems inconsistent with the notion that we can only hold seven items in our working memory. What is going on here, however, is that the constant repetition of the sequence enables us to use our long-term memories to complete the task; if the sequence was randomly generated in each round, we would come unstuck much earlier on.

■ On Brain Signals and Capacity

So what changes take place in the brain as children increase their capacity? In studies that my colleagues and I have been conducting at Karolinska Institutet over the past few years, children have been given simple tasks to perform involving remembering the position of dots, and have had their brain activity measured as they do so. Our findings suggest the presence of specific areas that increase their activity during childhood: one in the parietal lobe, one in the upper part of the frontal lobe, and one in the anterior part of the frontal lobe. This concurs with what other researchers have found.

The folds and creases of the parietal lobe, which is a rather large part of the brain, form a furrow called the intraparietal sulcus, and it is around this sulcus that we have observed the most distinct changes. This is exactly the same spot where previous studies have registered activity during tasks of controlled attention.

Which area of the frontal lobe is activated differently in children and adults depends on the task in hand. Numerous studies have noted such variances in the same upper area of the frontal lobe as is active in the control of attention. When working memory tasks include distracters, we also see differences in activity in the prefrontal cortex. These three areas can thus all be linked to capacity: higher activity is associated with better memory.

Another way of finding key structures that limit working memory is to take the capacity limitation curve reproduced in the introduction (see page 9) and search for brain areas whose activity resembles that described by the curve.

Two studies published in *Nature* in 2004 did just this. In the one study, subjects had to keep two, four, six, or eight different items—in this case the color and position of small circles displayed on a screen—in their working memory. It was found that performance on this task gradually wanes in exactly the same way as the graph predicts. fMRI was then used to measure brain activity, upon which one, and only one, brain area was found to match the appearance of the capacity curve. The area was in the intraparietal sulcus. The other study analyzed electrical activity using EEG and again found one area matching the curve—again, the intraparietal sulcus.

So what about problem-solving ability, which is thought to be linked to working memory capacity? In one large-scale study led by Kun Ho Lee at Seoul National University, scientists measured the performance of young people on Raven's matrices and then measured their brain activity as they carried out working memory tasks. A correlation between their problem-solving ability and brain activity was registered in both the parietal and frontal lobes, most notably in the sulcus intraparietalis—the very same place that my team and others have found correlates closely with the development of working memory capacity during childhood.

So as we can see, numerous studies indicate that it is areas of the parietal and frontal lobes that determine our working memory capacity. Rather than there being nebulous differences spread across the brain, there is a rather small number of well-defined areas—the same ones that we now know are active when information is retained in working memory and when the spotlight of attention is directed on a predetermined spot. Perhaps it is here where we will find the key structures, or bottleneck, that restricts our ability to receive and retain information. That the frontal lobe would be involved was perhaps to be expected, since for decades the area has been loosely linked to higher cognitive functions. However, the discovery that the parietal lobe is important to problem-solving and working memory is relatively new. The fact that a wide range of studies using different approaches so unequivocally point toward the parietal lobe is also quite noteworthy.

It was possibly no coincidence that it was the parietal lobe that was so singular about Einstein's brain. His brain was no larger or heavier than other brains; it did not have richer connections between the hemispheres, more neurons per square inch, or significantly bigger frontal lobes. The parietal lobes, however, were quite distinctive: not only were they much broader than in other brains, they were also asymmetrical, the left lobe being much larger than the right. They also had a very special anatomy, in that the furrow that normally divides the parietal lobe had an anterior

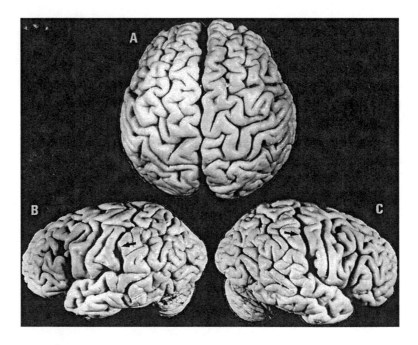

FIGURE 5-2
Einstein's brain. The arrows indicate the more anterior sulci (from Witelson et al., 1999).

displacement, which has been interpreted as the result of an early childhood expansion of this part of the cortex.

■ Mechanisms of Capacity Limitation

Let us assume that we have identified the key cortical areas responsible for the development of mental capacity during childhood. What happens in these areas of the parietal and frontal lobes when the information load rises? Why do these areas not have boundless capacity? Several studies have looked at changes in brain activity when the number of letters, digits, or faces that subjects have to remember is increased, and have generated a fair amount of consensus that blood flow and metabolism gradually escalate in direct proportion to the amount of information. Could this mean that there is some kind of metabolic limit to brain work that restricts the supply of oxygen or blood to the relevant brain areas, and that it is this that imposes limits on working memory? Maybe lactic acid builds up in the brain? If you have ever done a working memory test in which you hear a series of digits that you then have to repeat in reverse order, the idea of lactic acid in the brain might not seem too unreasonable.

However, none of these explanations seems particularly likely. For one, the brain's blood supply makes sure that the nerve cells always receive enough oxygenated blood. In fact, when nerve cells are activated and step up their metabolism and oxygen consumption, the blood flow to that particular area rises so much that it overcompensates, and supplies the cells with more oxygen and blood than they have when resting. We also know that in certain extreme circumstances, such as during an epileptic seizure, the blood flow to the brain can be very much higher than when people do demanding mental tasks. We will have to look for other possible explanations. Can we, for instance, look at what happens in the cerebral cortices of the parietal and frontal lobes during childhood development to understand the mechanisms behind improved working memory?

■ The Child's Brain

Studies of children's brains can repudiate the least sophisticated idea of what makes a highly functional brain: one with many nerve cells. There are almost twice as many interneuronal connections (synapses) in the frontal lobes of a two-year-old as there are in those of a twenty-year-old, yet the two-year-old has a much poorer working memory. From the age of two, synaptic density gradually decreases, reaching the adult level somewhere around the age of twelve. After a period of early overproduction, neurons, connectors, and synapses disappear with alarming speed. The fiber system connecting the two cerebral hemispheres loses 900,000 axons per day during the first three months. It is difficult to explain why capacity should increase when neurons disappear, but it is conceivable that the reinforcement of important connections and the deterioration of unimportant connections combine to improve the structure of the network.

Connecting nerve fibers are covered with a lipid sheath called myelin, which helps to amplify the speed of nerve impulses. During development, this myelin sheath thickens (myelinization); even though most myelinization takes places before the age of two, we now know that the brain continues the process up to early adulthood. MR studies have also been able to link the myelinization of connections between the parietal and frontal lobes with the development of working memory. Just why this should lead to a better working memory is by no means self-evident. One possibility is that it is the result of faster connections; another is that the myelin makes the connections more secure, so an impulse originating in the parietal lobe is more likely to be conveyed all the way to the frontal lobe.

There are thus a number of processes taking place in the child's brain as its capacity develops: the reinforcement of certain synaptic connections, the weakening of others, the decimation of links between different parts of the brain, and the myelinization of the links that remain. It is possible that the techniques now available to us for studying the human brain are too imprecise to answer the question of capacity limitation. The cause could be found, for instance, in the pattern of connections between individual neurons. Mischievous tongues sometimes compare brain imaging techniques such as PET and fMRI to measuring the temperature of a computer: you can detect a difference in temperature between when the computer is off and when it is on, and even possibly find differences between its components, but you will still be light-years away from understanding its workings.

■ Computer Simulation of Brain Activity

It is hoped that one day scientists will be able to combine high-resolution methods, such as electrophysiology, by which we can see the activity of individual neurons with the help of ultrafine needles, with brain imagery techniques that allow us to measure that activity of several brain areas simultaneously, and thus integrate macroscopic and microscopic information. We might also learn enough about neurons and their connections to be able to build realistic computer models of the brain, which we could then use to test different hypotheses of how neurons behave. My own research group is engaged in such a project with Jesper Tegnér, Fredrik Edin, and Julian Macoveanu, who are devising computer models of working memory in order to understand the neuronal development that accounts for the increase in brain capacity and the changes in brain activity that occur during childhood.

We have used in our studies a network of about a hundred virtual nerve cells, which in the brain would correspond to less than one square millimeter of the frontal cortex. We have calibrated the network so that the activity resembles that previously recorded in primates when retaining information in working memory. Such a tiny network can also retain information in its "working memory"; what's more, just as we have observed in monkeys, this information is stored through continual neuronal activity during the delay period and kept fresh by a process of feedback.

So what does this model tell us about how we can improve capacity? In one experiment we tested two hypotheses: that it is *stronger connections* between nerve cells that gives us a better working memory, or that it is *faster connections* (i.e., the more efficient transmission of an impulse from one brain area to another) that improves capacity. The latter method would depend on myelinization, and was my favorite hypothesis since MR studies have previously shown that the myelinization of certain areas of the brain is linked to the development of working memory.

A "child model network" and an "adult model network" were built for each hypothesis. We then stimulated the networks and measured their activity as they retained information in their "working memories." We also measured brain activity using fMRI in children and adults to see which hypothesis best fit the data.

It turned out that the first hypothesis was superior. A network of stronger synapses was more stable and able to retain mnemonic activity even when subjected to disturbance. The activity of the network also matched our fMRI observations. To my disappointment, my favorite hypothesis, involving faster connections, did not seem able to explain the changes in brain activity recorded in the experiment.

I began this book by asking which functions limit mental powers when the Stone Age brain meets the information flood. It seemed that the capacity of working memory was one of the principal bottlenecks. When we then looked around the brain to find where this bottleneck was located, we discovered that working memory capacity is not spread diffusely across the entire neocortex but instead linked to a few key areas in the parietal and frontal lobes. When we took yet another step and asked which mechanisms limit the capacity of these areas, we started to approach the front line of current research and found ourselves, for the time being, without any clear answers. Computer simulations suggest that it might have something to do with stronger synaptic connections between neurons.

In the next chapter, we will be returning to the information flood and some of the mentally demanding everyday situations that really put our information-processing skills to the test, such as when we have to do a job in the face of distractions or when we try to multitask. Previously, we have seen that working memory capacity is of critical importance to a number of mental tasks. Is it the same capacity and the same key areas of the brain that determine our ability to handle distractions and simultaneous tasks? Why is it sometimes so hard for our brains to do two things at once?

6 ■

Simultaneous Capacity and
Mental Bandwidth

Multi-tasking has long been a well-known strategy adopted by the overperforming and the impatient for getting more things done more quickly.

Some simultaneous tasks, such as shaving while having breakfast, are difficult for motor reasons. Others, such as reading a map while driving, can be difficult because we can take in information from only one source and direct our gaze to only one thing at a time. Yet others are difficult to do simultaneously because they require the similar processing of information somewhere between input and output, between stimulus and response. In many cases, both tasks put demands on working memory. According to Michael Posner, the results of numerous studies in this field can be reduced, rather simplistically, to the graph in Figure 6.1.

According to this model, performance will always lie somewhere along this curve. If task A is reading the paper and task B is talking to your other half at the breakfast table, you can choose, for example, to concentrate on the

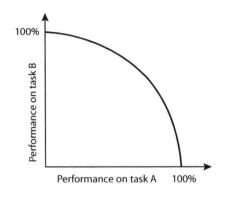

FIGURE 6-1
Performance on simultaneous tasks (from Posner, 1978).

news and ignore your partner (do not try this experiment at home). Your performance on A will then be 100 percent (by definition) and 0 percent on B. If you then start to listen to your partner and give a few cursory responses, you will start moving up the curve. Your performance on B will improve sharply from 0, but your reading will be a little slower and you will find yourself having to reread the more difficult passages: your performance on task A is beginning to wane. If you put your paper down and give your partner your undivided attention, you will be performing 100 percent on task B and 0 percent on task A.

Going by the graph, in performing task A to 90 percent of our ability, we would be carrying out task B to about 44 percent. So suddenly we would have increased our work capacity to 134 percent of what it would have been had we done the two tasks consecutively. Part of the reason for this is that we can quickly switch between the two tasks and sacrifice a certain degree of efficiency. The other factor that we have to take into consideration is the price we pay for executing a task at 90 percent of our capacity instead of 100 percent. If you answer wrongly when asked if you want milk in your coffee or have to reread a sentence, this price is not so high, and it's often no problem picking up a ball that you drop while trying to keep many balls in the air at once. There are instances, however, when we make decisions and don't get a chance to pick up that dropped ball. You should not, for example, decide where to invest your pension savings while trying to plow through that morning's headlines, or conduct a job interview while reading your e-mails.

When people discuss simultaneous performance, it is never long before someone makes the following two claims: that women are better than men at dual-tasking, and that this is due to the thickness of the connection between the two cerebral hemispheres. "Women have broadband in their heads" is a phrase that has become something of a mantra. However, there is no support for this in the literature on systematic gender differences. For example, in a review conducted by Merrill Hiscock at the University of Houston, only 4 out of 112 experiments found evidence for general differences in dual-task interference: two favored men, two favored women. It is true that there are differences in the shape and thickness of the corpus callosum (the scientific name for the bundle of nerve fibers connecting the left and right brain hemispheres), but just what functional significance this has for dual-task performance nobody knows. The superior dual-task ability of women is clearly just an urban legend.

■ Driving and Talking on the Phone

Studies of everyday activities, such as cleaning, conversing, or driving, are difficult to do because the activities vary so much from one moment to the next. Driving a car along a seemingly endless straight stretch of highway requires fewer decisions than trying to find your way though a city center; conversing can involve passive listening or more cognitively demanding discussions. One way of studying dual-tasking while driving is therefore to do it in the laboratory, where the task can be simulated and specific cognitive tasks given to the driver to perform simultaneously.

In one study of dual-tasking while driving, it was shown that performance was not impaired by listening to the radio or an audiobook. However, more cognitively demanding tasks, such as holding a discussion, did interfere with driving and not only caused subjects to miss simulated traffic lights twice as often but also slowed down their reaction times. In fact, the effect of cell phone conversations is comparable to driving with a blood alcohol level above the legal limit; the Human Factors and Ergonomics Society estimates that 2,600 deaths and 330,000 injuries are caused each year in the United States by motorists speaking on their cell phones while driving.

Another study of dual-tasking specifically investigated how it relates to working memory. The researchers used a car simulator in the form of half a Saab 9000 with a projector screen instead of a windshield to create the impression of driving along a highway. All the subjects were asked to do was to keep a reasonable distance from the car ahead and to brake when it did. The task was first performed without any other simultaneous task. The researchers then tested the subjects' dual-tasking abilities by asking them to drive while memorizing and repeating words that were read out to them. In this situation, reaction times were half a second slower than when they only had the road to concentrate on. With people over sixty, who have poorer working memory capacity, they found even more dramatic effects—a delay of roughly one and a half seconds in reaction time when the load on working memory was high.

So some of the limitations on dual-tasking have to do with working memory. In a later chapter, we will be taking a look at the brain structure that imposes this limit. First, however, let us consider a situation that closely resembles dual-tasking: performing under distraction.

◼ The Cocktail Party Effect and Other Distractions

When Linda is sitting reading a report in her open-plan office while trying to listen in on her neighbor's telephone conversation, she is effectively dual-tasking. If, instead, she decides to focus exclusively on her reading and to shut out the telephone conversation and other surrounding distracters, we have a distraction situation. All irrelevant information, such as her neighbor's conversation, now constitutes distracting stimuli that she must try to ignore.

The balance between working memory demands and distraction was the subject of a series of experiments by, among others, London-based psychologists Nilli Lavie and Jan de Fockert. They demonstrated that when people perform tasks that load working memory, and thus place heavy demands on their mental capacity, they become more easily distracted. They were also able to show that the degree of distraction correlates with the level of activity in the part of the brain that encodes the distractions.

Similar conclusions have been drawn by a study carried out by Edward Vogel and his research group at the University of Oregon. In one paper they demonstrated that people with higher working memory capacity are better at ignoring distractions. They also used a method of measuring how the electrical activity of the parietal lobe changes with the information load of working memory. Using this technique, they were able to show that people with lower working memory capacity were unable to distinguish between relevant and irrelevant information. Put another way, we could say that as they store information about the distracters in working memory, irrelevant information occupies space in the brain that should have been reserved for relevant information.

One question raised by Vogel's study was how this filtering is controlled. In order to find out, my colleague Fiona McNab and I performed a study where subjects a received a cue a few seconds before the working memory trial informing them whether the trial would contain distracters that should be filtered out or whether they should remember all the information that was presented to them. We found that such an instructional cue resulted in increased brain activity in the prefrontal cortex and in the basal ganglia, a gray-matter structure deeper down in the brain. This activity predicted how good subjects later were at filtering out irrelevant information. These structures thus seemed able to control access to working memory storage—acting as, so to speak, "the brain's spam filter." Moreover, subjects with higher working memory capacity had higher activity in these areas.

A well-known example of distractibility is the "cocktail party effect." When you are standing in the middle of a group of chatting people, you still have the ability to concentrate on the one to whom you are talking. You direct the spotlight of your attention at him or her, which enables you to filter out all the other conversations going on around you. But sometimes, such as when someone behind you mentions your name, you cannot help being distracted, and your attention is drawn away from your conversational partner and toward the possible gossip.

This can be seen as an example of the balance between the controlled attention system and the stimulus-driven attention system. The controlled system directs your attention to the person to whom you are talking, while the stimulus-driven system draws your attention to other stimuli around you.

What psychologists have recently discovered is that people differ in how they perform in the cocktail party situation: while some continue to keep their attention fixed on the relevant conversation despite the overheard name-dropping, about one in three find themselves distracted. It turns out that what separates the two groups is working memory, in that those with the lowest working memory capacity are also the most easily distracted. This also agrees with what we found earlier in this book: that we need working memory to control our attention. When our working memory fails us, the distractions and the stimulus-driven system take over. Another example of this is the fact that people with lower working memory capacity often fail to attend to the task at hand, and instead spend more time "mind wandering." This was shown in a study by Michael Kane and colleagues at the University of North Carolina. They gave PDAs to their subjects, and when an alarm from the PDA went off, which happended eight times a day, the subjects would immediately fill out a questionnaire of what they had been doing, and whether they were concentrating on the task at hand, or if their mind had been wandering. What they found was that as soon as tasks became mentally challenging, the subjects with lower working memory capacity also displayed a higher degree of mind-wandering.

Linda's success at shutting out the outside world will thus be determined by two factors: how mentally demanding her task is and how much distraction, or how strong, there is around her. How demanding the task is depends, in turn, on how much information she has to keep in her working memory and her working memory capacity.

Linda's working memory capacity might be influenced by her mood or state of mind: if she has a baby at home who keeps her awake at night, it will be impaired by the lack of sleep, so the task will appear harder and the distractions more distracting. Further, the working memory load can be determined by the difficulty of the text, in that a text containing long sentences and difficult words is more demanding.

What we find in situations like this is that working memory performance and distractions are placed on either side of a pair of scales, and the balance determines the probability of our succeeding with our demanding working memory task. If we have a lot of distractions around us, we need good working memory capacity to manage the task. So if we have a lot of information in our working memory, we are more distraught than when we have a little. The greater level of distraction associated with the modern information technology society thus places higher demands on our working memory.

Cell phones are fantastic, but they also place us in a "cocktail party situation," in which we have to ignore irrelevant speech, all day long. In another example, open-plan offices improve communication between employees, but the greater disturbance this causes also requires more of our working memories.

■ What Happens in the Brain When We Do Two Things at Once?

What is it about the way the brain is organized that means that we sometimes fail and sometimes manage, fairly well

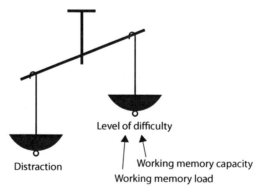

FIGURE 6-2
An example of the interaction between distraction, working memory capacity and working memory load.

at that, to do two things at once? In the psychological literature, it has been suggested that dual-tasking would require an extra function, which is sometimes referred to as the "central executive"—the very same module that psychologist Alan Baddeley posits as the "coordinating factor" in working memory. But is it possible to find any central executive in the brain? Some scientists maintain that it is. Mark D'Esposito and his group measured brain activity first as their subjects performed tasks consecutively and again when they performed them simultaneously. Doing this, they found that there were some areas, including in the frontal lobe, that were activated only when subjects were performing two tasks simultaneously and not when they performed them one at a time. This, they concluded, was the neurological equivalent of the central executive, a separate module for coordinating and monitoring activity taking place elsewhere in the brain.

The term "central executive" has, however, been criticized for conjuring up the image of some little man in the brain, a homunculus that sits there directing things. The problem with this is what then directs the activity of *his* brain when *he* has to do two things at once—an even smaller homunculus?

An alternative hypothesis for why two tasks are not always doable at once is that they both demand access to the same brain area. The performance of a task is hardly ever linked to just one brain area; rather, it is associated with a network of areas. If we now imagine two networks, A and B, that require access to the same area at the same time, we can see that this causes a conflict: either the activity will alternate between that of network A and that of network B, which deprives both areas of full access to the area, or the networks will be active simultaneously but will not be fully effective because they interfere with each other in the overlap. We could, if we so wished, describe it by saying that the capacity of the area is exceeded.

There are thus two different hypotheses on how concurrent performance and working memory are related. Hypothesis 1 is that concurrent performance requires an extra, superior center that coordinates the activity in the two networks involved. To explain why two tasks are performed less well than one task, we must also assume that this center does not execute its coordinating responsibilities perfectly. Hypothesis 2 (the overlap hypothesis) is that two tasks interfere with each other because they both need to use the same cortical area at the same time. The cause of this interference, then, is in the same brain system that deals with working memory.

To test these hypotheses, my colleagues and I had subjects carry out a visual working memory task, an auditory working memory task, or both simultaneously. We measured the blood flow in their brains and looked for anything that might corroborate either of the hypotheses. We found no extra area in the brain that was only activated when the tasks were performed simultaneously. There was, however, an overlap between the two networks, which supports hypothesis 2. In another study, we also observed that the more the brain activity for the two tasks overlapped, the more they interfere with each other.

There is a complicated simultaneous task that psychologists often like to use and that reveals a very high correlation between performance and success on tests of reading

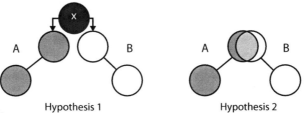

Hypothesis 1   Hypothesis 2

FIGURE 6-3
Two hypotheses on how the brain handles simultaneous situations.

comprehension. In this task, subjects hear a series of statements to which they have to answer true or false. They also have to remember the last word of each statement so that they can repeat them at the end of the experiment. If, for example, you hear the following statements:

Dogs can swim
Frogs have ears
Airplanes are lighter than air
Arms have knees
Birds can fly

you are to answer true to the first statement and keep the word *swim* in your working memory, then answer false to the next one and keep both the words *swim* and *ears* in your working memory, and so forth. When you have five different words in your working memory and try to respond to the sixth statement, you really start to feel the load on your working memory.

In one study that I conducted with Silvia Bunge and John Gabrieli at Stanford University, we studied brain activity during this dual task. We found, again, that there was no extra area concomitant with those activated when the students responded to statements or remembered words. To be sure, the frontal lobe was activated more during the simultaneous task, but we saw no additional brain area that was *not* activated during one of the individual tasks.

So our simultaneous experiment contradicted hypothesis 1. Results from a group at Yale University including Patricia Goldman-Rakic also supported our findings, and found no extra area during the simultaneous task. However, more recent research has breathed new life into attempts to find a special area of the brain that handles concurrent performance during more complex tasks requiring switching between tasks A and B while keeping information from both tasks in working memory when the switching is done in a random and unpredictable way. The jury is therefore still out on this; however, the fact that there is an overlap is sufficient to explain why two simultaneous tasks interfere with each other, regardless of whether or not an extra area is also sometimes engaged.

How well we manage to multi-task can therefore often be related to the information load on working memory. Often we can do the tasks if one of them is automatic, such as walking; we can usually manage that quite well while carrying out other tasks that occupy working memory. Usually, for an activity to be designated "automatic," it no longer demands any activation of the frontal lobes. However, a working memory task can never be automatic, as the information it contains always has to be encoded through the continual activation of the frontal and parietal lobes. This can be why it is so difficult to do two working memory tasks at once.

■ The Unifying Capacity Hypothesis

Overlapping areas of the neocortex will form a kind of information-processing bottleneck; consequently, the constraints imposed on our simultaneous abilities might be attributable to capacity limitations in a handful of brain areas. What is really interesting is that the overlaps that have been observed in the simultaneous experiments—in the parietal and frontal lobes—are the same, in part, as those identified as being crucial to working memory capacity.

We saw from different psychological experiments how working memory capacity was fundamental to our ability to dual-task and to how well we are able to shut out distracting information. In preceding chapters, we saw how this capacity develops during childhood, how it differs in adults, and how it seemed to be determined by a number of key areas—in the intraparietal sulcus and the frontal lobes. And we saw that research into simultaneous tasks points at these very same bottleneck areas for our simultaneous abilities.

There are, of course, a great many simultaneous situations that I have left untouched in this chapter, such as our inability to react to two different but almost concurrent stimuli (the telephone and the doorbell ringing at the same time) or to perform two complex motor tasks at once (running and juggling or rubbing your stomach and patting your head, for example), in which our limitations have nothing to do with working memory. But for most cognitively demanding tasks, it seems as if two separate phenomena—constraints on working memory and constraints on simultaneous abilities—can be attributed to the same mechanism: the limited capacity of the overlap areas, or key areas, in the parietal and frontal lobes. In many cases, our simultaneous capacity and our ability to handle distractions seem reducible to working memory capacity. We have thus identified some of the bottlenecks of the Stone Age brain, areas that determine our ability to handle the information flood.

In the next chapter, instead of probing more deeply into neurons and fMRI studies, we will be shedding light on the problem of the Stone Age brain and the information flood from another angle by taking a look at different theories of how this capacity originally came about. When discussing the brain's limitations and potential, it is not unreasonable to examine the conditions under which its capacity first developed. Perhaps the most striking question is not why there is some sort of upper limit to our ability to handle information but why this ability evolved in the first place. The digital information age in which we now find ourselves seems to lay claim to all our resources and a little more, but the brains with which we are born are, genetically speaking, little different from those that Cro-Magnons were born with some forty thousand years ago. What sense can be made of this?

7 ■
Wallace's Paradox

In 1858, Charles Darwin received a letter from a young explorer named Alfred R. Wallace. In it, Wallace described an idea about the origin of species that he had developed completely independently of Darwin while he lay in a malarial fever on a small island in the Malaysian archipelago. Darwin was shocked at the similarity with his own as yet unpublished theories, and the letter made him hasten the publication of his own manuscript, which came out the following year.

Wallace and Darwin were to exchange their thoughts on evolution for several years. In many respects, their opinions were the same, but they also disagreed on certain points of theory; most notably, Wallace could never accept any principle other than adaptivity—which is to say that evolution is driven by the optimal adaptation of species to their surroundings for their survival.

Darwin proposed other possibilities, including sexual selection, by which certain species characteristics are reinforceable only because they give an advantage for mating, not because they have any immediate survival value. The tail feathers of the peacock are a typical example of sexual selection. They have developed through a process of evolution, but because they supply no advantage when flying or feeding, for instance, they offer no adaptation to the environment in which the birds live. The only advantage lies in the fact that as peahens show a preference for decorative tail feathers, well-endowed peacocks will reproduce more than their rivals, thus driving evolution toward larger and more elaborate tails.

The greatest conundrum that faced Wallace with the extreme adaptivity of humans was the development of the brain. In many respects he was unusual for his time in that he believed that natives of primitive societies had brains that were in no way inferior to those of contemporary European philosophers and mathematicians. This he based, in part, on comparisons of size. However, somehow this did not really fit with the apparently simple lives that natives led: how could evolution give early man this extreme surplus of intellectual capacity? In Wallace's own words:

> A brain slightly larger than that of the gorilla would . . . fully have sufficed for the limited mental development of the savage; and we must therefore admit, that the large brain he actually possesses could never have been solely developed by any of those laws of evolution, whose essence is, that they lead to a degree of organization exactly proportionate to the wants of each species, never beyond those wants.

Wallace would never solve this paradox, and had to resort to divine intervention as an explanation. He believed that everything on the planet had evolved through natural selection and adaptation—apart from the human brain, that is, which could only have been created by a god. Scientists have since developed alternative explanations that we ought to consider before turning religious.

■ The Evolution of Working Memory

Despite the tiny genetic changes that have been taking place continually over time, the similarities between the Cro-Magnon brain and the brain of a human today are much, much greater than the differences. The size of the brain has not changed for forty thousand years, and any slight genetic modifications cannot explain the technological and cultural developments that have occurred at this end of the evolutionary time line. If we want to attribute

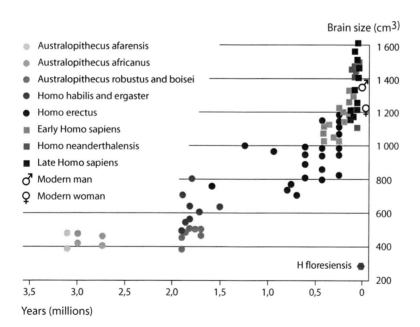

FIGURE 7-1
Brain size of early hominids and modern humans (from Dunbar, 1996).

innate faculties to adaptations to a specific environment, we must therefore look back into the mists of time.

When speculating about what took place forty thousand years ago, the discussion becomes necessarily fuzzier. Nor is there much to glean from the literature specifically on the evolution of working memory. I will therefore broaden the discussion a little and talk more generally about theories of the development of intelligence, looking at the extent to which they are applicable to working memory.

A qualified guess as to why cognitive capacity developed is that it was needed for social interaction. Even Darwin was proposing that human intelligence evolved as an adaptation to collective living. Evolutionary psychologist Robin Dunbar from the University of Liverpool has also shown that in primates, the ratio of cortical size to total brain size is proportional to the size of the group in which the animal naturally congregates. The larger the cortex, the larger the social group. If this law also applied to humans, it would suggest a natural social group of around 150 individuals, which seems to tally with some estimations of how large the groups, or clans, were during the hunter-gatherer era—even though most of that time was spent in smaller clusters.

But how exactly would working memory be needed for social interaction? Perhaps it came in handy for understanding interactions between other humans and their interests, or simply for purloining food or mates from others in the group in a "He thinks that I think that he thinks . . ." kind of way—a game that can become quite complex. Psychologists Richard Byrne and Andrew Whiten from the University of St. Andrews have developed a theory on the role of the social game in cerebral development, and coined the term "Machiavellian intelligence," with reference to the Italian writer and politician, who taught the art of dominion through manipulation. Such a person, one could say, looks upon his or her social environment in much the same way as a chess player looks upon a chess board, with all the planning and prediction that the game involves.

Another possible reason for the growth of intelligence and working memory is the development of language. Language requires a symbolic representation of whatever it is we want to express; we must also be able to hold together the different parts of a sentence if we are to understand it. So it might not come as too much of a surprise to find that working memory capacity correlates highly with reading comprehension. It was arguably the development of language that led to a technological revolution some forty thousand years ago. It was at the end of this evolutionary spurt that we see some of the earliest paintings in the caves of Cro-Magnon in southwest France, more advanced tools such as hooks and barbed spears, and, later, the appearance of representational artifacts.

With language, early hominids could plan, cooperate, and pass on knowledge in ways that had not been possible previously. The more complex environment that they created around them also necessitated a more complex language. In *The Symbolic Species*, Terrence Deacon argues that language thus evolved through a process of feedback with technology and culture.

Dunbar, on the other hand, preferred to dwell upon how linguistic development went hand in hand with that of the social environment and the extended community. Living in a group requires the maintaining of friendships. In a colony of chimpanzees this can be achieved by plucking fleas off each other. When the size of the group exceeds a certain threshold, grooming is no longer a viable option. What Dunbar suggests is that language, or rather "gossip," fulfilled the function that flea picking once did, making the primary purpose of language social bonding. Moreover, large groups are required in order to obtain the large number of individuals needed to develop and nurture a language. It follows, then, that language was both a consequence and a precondition of extended community living.

A more unusual explanation for the development of intelligence is sexual selection, so that rather than having any survival value, intelligence evolved out of a need to impress the opposite sex and exhibit the quality of one's genes—in much the same way as the peacock's beautiful but perfectly useless tail feathers do. This is a theory advocated by evolutionary psychologist Geoffrey Miller at the University of New Mexico, who argues that activities with no overt survival value, such as dance, music, and art, developed as a display of intelligence and genetic superiority to the opposite sex. Miller also conjectures that this might also explain why so many young people dream of becoming rock stars.

■ Intelligence as a By-product

Attempts to understand our mental abilities from hypotheses about the way early humans lived appeal to and fire the imagination. Evolutionary psychology has also enjoyed much popularity in recent times, thanks in part to the books of Steven Pinker. The problem with such theories is they are virtually impossible to prove and equally impossible to disprove. What we know of prehistoric societies we learn from stones and bones. How they talked, thought, and organized their communities we have no idea. Of course, we can make assumptions to explain whatever we like, but they are assumptions nonetheless. To be sure, the social game can be formulated in terms of problems that require working memory. But how do we quantify social complexity two hundred thousand or forty thousand years ago? Linguistic communication demands working memory, but just how complicated were the utterances of the Upper Paleolithic era?

Paleontologist and evolutionary theorist Stephen Jay Gould launched some of the fiercest attacks on evolutionary psychology. One of his arguments is that evolutionary psychological theory can explain any aspect of human development, but does so by making a number of arbitrary assumptions. However, the main problem with evolutionary psychology as he sees it is that it is based on a rigid belief in adaptation, the supposition being that all our innate faculties are a collection of tools that were built up by way of optimal adaptation to some particular demands of mankind's childhood. It was just this that led Wallace into his paradox. However, according to Gould this is a logical fallacy, and not even Darwin suggested that adaptation was the sole mechanism driving the evolution of species.

Evolution through sexual selection is an alternative to exclusively adaptive evolution. Gould also raises the possibility that an organ fulfills a particular function during one phase of evolution but then starts to be used for some other purpose during another. The body is also full of evolutionary by-products that may not even have been functional when they appeared but also may not have cost so much to keep. We know, for example, that a genetic mutation often causes not one but several changes; if one of these changes has a survival value while the others are survival-neutral, all of them may be retained simply by virtue of their association with the same mutation.

Gould gives many examples of developmental and evolutionary by-products, including everything from male nipples to the panda's thumb. This latter is a tiny bone in the panda's hand called the radial sesamoid. In humans, it is smaller than a pea; in the panda, it has developed into something resembling an extra thumb that can be used when paring leaves and shoots from bamboo plants. The panda has a similar growth, albeit shorter, by the corresponding sesamoid bone of the foot. This bone, however, is totally without function. It is likely that the evolution of both protuberances is linked, in that the same genetic mutations caused the growth of the sesamoid bones of both extremities. One of these mutations—that in the hand—was functional, and because of this both mutations were preserved. The other—the one in the foot—is an evolutionary mutation that has no function: a by-product. It is therefore a mistake to assume that each organ is perfectly developed to perform a certain function and then to search for this function in our evolutionary history. The body is full of nonadaptive phenomena, argues Gould, perhaps none more so than the brain. One example could be the highly specialized parts of the cortex that we use for reading, areas that could not have evolved as an optimal adaptation to text in our environment.

As for the brain, a genetic mutation might well have caused the overdevelopment of several areas of the cortex. All it would have taken is for one of these areas to have been used for a purpose that provided greater survival value during a critical period of our evolution for the change to have been preserved. The other areas affected by the same genetic mutation might not have proved useful until thousands of years later.

Gould's criticism of evolutionary theory appeals to the scientific skepticism of many, including myself. The idea that the brain is full of by-products implies that it is also full of undreamed-of possibilities, which is a wonderful thought.

To recap, then: Evolutionary psychological theories attribute the development of our intelligence, and possibly our working memory, to our social environment, our language, and the development of a complex culture. Other theories put it down to sexual selection or by-productism. A combination of different ideas is also feasible, of course.

It could be the case that evolution has provided us with an area of the brain that is able to retain and manipulate symbolic representations in working memory. One such brain area might once have had survival value in that it endowed us with the potential to learn a language or handle social situations. If this area was multimodal, however, and could thus hold symbolic representations in working memory irrespective of whether they were linguistic or visual, we would have been able to use the same area to devise new traps in which to catch prey—or, thousands of years later, to work out differential equations and solve Raven's matrices.

If we adopt a strict adaptationist evolutionary perspective and see working memory as a tool genetically adapted to the particular demands of the environment in which we lived forty thousand years ago, we have a problem in that the environments with which we have to cope today are much more complex and demanding, and increasingly so. This is Wallace's paradox applied to the question of what happens when the Stone Age brain meets the information flood. One way out of this paradox is the assumptions that our mental faculty developed either as a by-product or through sexual selection and thus bestowed on us an over-capacity at some early stage of our development.

Another possibility—and this is the joker in the pack—is the brain's plasticity. It is true that, genetically speaking, we are pretty much identical to Cro-Magnons, but how much of our brain capacity is nature and how much is nurture? To what extent are we born with a set of finished tools, and to what extent are our tools fashioned after birth?

8 ∎

Brain Plasticity

In earlier chapters, we identified a number of potential key areas for our working memory capacity, and laid them out on the brain map. The cognitive neurosciences, which saw a burst of popularity in the 1990s along with the development of new brain imaging techniques, have largely been devoted to this very kind of mapping, in which different areas of the brain are assigned different functions. Sometimes the science is mocked, its detractors dismissing it as a kind of modern phrenology. The phrenologists were nineteenth-century charlatans who made pronouncements about human characteristics by feeling the depressions and bumps of the cranium. Not only were the phrenologists unscientific, but their measurements of the skull also fed into early-twentieth-century racial biology.

The association with phrenology is, however, rather simplistic. Vernon Mountcastle, one of the twentieth century's great neuroscientists, although never having engaged in brain imaging himself, was something of an apologist for phrenology. There were, he argued, two assumptions that phrenology made: first, that different functions were associated with different parts of the brain, and second, that the functions of these areas were proclaimed by the contours of the cranium. While the latter assumption is pure nonsense, the first actually turns out to be correct and is a theoretically crucial point.

One of the first studies demonstrating the localization of function was done by the French neurologist Paul Broca. Broca received a patient who had been struck by a sudden inability to talk, and when the patient died, Broca examined the man's brain and found a lesion in the left frontal lobe. This was the first time that an association between a specific function and an area of the brain had been demonstrated.

In the early 1900s, Korbinian Brodmann described regional differences in cell structure and constructed one of the first maps of the brain, which he divided into fifty-two separate areas, developing a nomenclature that is still used to this day.

Techniques such as PET and fMRI have permitted great strides to be made in functional topography. Scientists have also relinquished the somewhat simplified notion of one area, one function. Instead, it seems that each function is related to a network of areas and that one and the same area can be involved in multiple such networks. Nevertheless, the map fixation remains. Implicit in this topographical mind-set, however, is a kind of inert constancy: maps lay out immutable things—mountains and rivers are where they are. It is only recently that research has focused on the degree to which these maps can shift and change.

■ How the Brain Map Is Redrawn

That the brain is mutable is nothing new; indeed, it is self-evident. If a schoolgirl cannot define certain words on

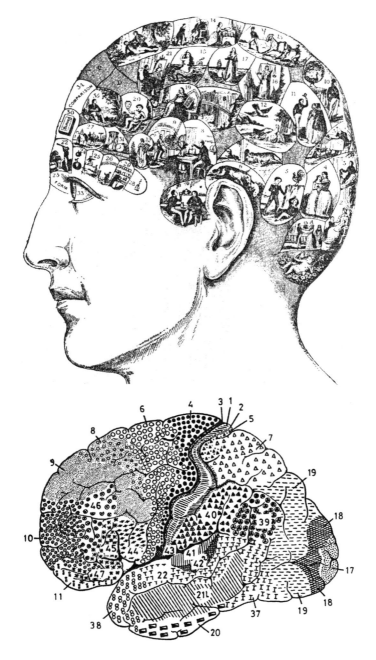

Figure 8-1A and B
A: The phrenologist's functional organization of the cranium.
B: Korbinian Brodmann's model of brain organization, based on differences in neuronal structure, was conceived in the early 20th century, and is still used to name the different parts of the brain.

Wednesday but goes home to study and on Thursday knows exactly what the word *phanerogam* means, her brain has altered slightly from the one day to the next. There is, after all, nowhere else to store the information (cheat notes excluded). However, it is of interest to see when, where, and how the brain changes.

As mentioned previously, much of our knowledge of how the functional map is redrawn comes from situations in which the brain is deprived of informational input. If a person loses a body part, so a sensory area of the brain no longer receives the corresponding information, surrounding parts of the brain will start to encroach on this area. If, for instance, signals are no longer conveyed from the index finger to the index-finger area of the neocortex, this area will start to shrink, and the adjacent area, the one that receives signals from the middle finger, will start to expand.

This is not a question of nerve cells migrating from one location to another. True, it is possible that new neurons can be formed in certain parts of the brain, but no one has yet shown that this might have a function in these areas of the neocortex. What happens first is a change in the structure of the nerve cells, with the formation of small processes and the loss of others. Attached to these processes are the synapses, which mediate the cell's contact with its neighbors. The change in processes and synapses brings about a corresponding change in the cell's function. When we then take a bird's-eye view of the brain, we find that parts of the area that originally received sensory impressions from the index finger can now be activated by sensory input from the middle finger. The map has been redrawn.

It is possibly this same mechanism that allows that visual cortices of blind people to be activated when they read Braille. However, the fact that the visual cortices are activated when blind people read Braille does not necessarily mean that they use these areas to analyze the sensory information, and exactly what these areas do in such circumstances is not fully understood. Perhaps their visual cortices are activated by some process of unconscious visualization.

One fundamental question is how mutable the different parts of the brain actually are. Are they programmed from birth to carry out a specific task, or is their functionality determined by the stimuli they receive? Is it heredity or environment, nature or nurture? One interesting contribution to this debate has been made by a group led by Mriganka Sur at the Massachusetts Institute of Technology. Using laboratory animals, they transplanted the nerves that conduct visual impressions into the brain so that they transmitted signals to the auditory area instead. This led to a reorganization of the auditory area that left it resembling that of the visual area. They also found that the input signals could actually be used, allowing the animals to utilize their auditory cortices to see when they moved around. No scientist believes categorically in either nature or nurture, but Sur's results show how important sensory stimuli are for determining how the brain is organized, which in turn underpins the importance of environment.

■ The Effect of Stimulation

The example above illustrates how the brain map is redrawn when a function disappears so as to deprive the brain of information. Another type of change is that caused by enhanced stimulation, as occurs when a particular faculty is deliberately trained. Our understanding of this type of plasticity has grown out of work done in the 1990s and so is still relatively fresh.

An example of this is how we can train our ability to detect differences in pitch. Primates can learn to perform a task that involves listening to two consecutive notes, deciding if they have the same pitch or not, and pressing a button to give their answer. A study carried out by Gregg

Recanzone and Michael Merzenich at the University of California, San Francisco, showed that although at first monkeys could do this only if the two notes were very different, after hundreds of trials over weeks of training, their performance progressively improved until they were able to distinguish between two notes of almost identical pitch. When the scientists then examined which nerve cells in the primary auditory area were activated as the monkeys performed the task, they found that the number of activated brain cells was much greater, and the cortical representation therefore much larger, than in control monkeys.

Similar experiments have also been carried out on monkeys as they learn to perform specific kind of forelimb movements. After several weeks' training on a simple dexterity task, it was found that the motor area corresponding to the finger used had become enlarged. The results of these experiments demonstrate that the map representing the localization of different functions is extremely changeable.

■ Music and Juggling

Several studies have looked at how the brain is affected by long periods of musical instrument practice. Most important for us, changes have been observed in relation to the training of motor skills, making, for example, the cortical area that receives sensory input from the left hand larger in string musicians than in other people. Sara Bengtsson and Fredrik Ullén at Karolinska Institutet have also demonstrated that the white-matter pathway that transmits motor signals is more developed in pianists, the degree of enlargement being proportional to how long they have been playing.

However, learning an instrument entails a very protracted influence on the brain. What about the effect of a shorter period of training in humans? In one study, subjects were asked to learn a particular sequence of finger movements: middle finger–little finger–ring finger–middle finger–index finger, and so on. At first, the learning curve was shallow and errors were common. After ten days of practice, however, they were able to reproduce the sequence quickly and perfectly. This coincided with a significant increase in activity in the primary motor cortex, the area that controls the muscles.

Another study that is often cited in discussions of human brain plasticity is the one of juggling mentioned in the introduction, which found that the volume of a part of the occipital lobe was affected by only three months of practice. This also demonstrates how a short period of training can manifest itself in changes large enough to be measured with the relative imprecision of an MR scanner. The fact that the changes then partly receded also shows how plasticity is a double-edged sword: passivity also affects the brain.

■ What Do We Mean by "Use" and "It"?

Research into training-based brain plasticity, such as the juggling study and the musician study, seems to confirm that rather hackneyed—for the brain researcher and psychologist, at least—axiom "Use it or lose it." True as it may be that the brain changes depending on how it is used, we should be careful not to generalize. The first question we should ask when we hear such assertions is what "use" actually means. Are all kinds of activity equivalent? To draw an analogy with the body, we know that activity is generally good for us, and that the leg muscles waste away when the leg is in a cast after a break. At the same time, there is a difference between the daily use of our legs during a day in the office and what we subject our thigh muscles to doing leg presses in the gym. What type, intensity, and length of mental exercise are needed for it to have an effect?

There is most likely a vast difference between low-impact use and intense training.

Something we should also remember is that "Use it or lose it" does notrefer to the entire brain, but rather to specific functions and brain areas. If you practice discriminating between pitches, it is the auditory areas that will change, not those of the frontal or occipital lobes. Again, we can draw a parallel with physical exercise. If you extend and flex the right arm while holding a heavy dumbbell, you will build your right biceps, provided that the weight is heavy enough, you repeat the movement enough times, and you keep going for several weeks. But to say that this one exercise "develops the body" or "is good for the body" is a misleadingly vague statement.

In string musicians it was the sensory cortex representing the left hand that was enlarged, not that corresponding to the right hand. If you practice juggling, it is a specific area involved in the visual perception of movement that is affected.

The common interpretation of "Use it or lose it" is that "It is good for the brain to . . . " However, the fact that training a certain activity has an effect on the brain does not necessarily mean that it provides general exercise for the brain or generally strengthens mental capacity. Specific functions develop specific areas.

In the preceding chapter we suggested a possible solution to the paradox of how the Stone Age brain handles the information flood, namely, that the brain is able to adapt itself to its environment and the greater demands it entails. As we have seen in this chapter, there are plenty of examples showing how the brain can adapt to suit its environment and can be shaped by training. There is no reason that such plasticity should not also be possible in the frontal and parietal lobes, including the key areas that are associated with working memory capacity. It should, therefore, be theoretically feasible to develop working memory.

While such plasticity could take place passively, as an adaptation to living in a particular environment, it could also be exploited through the conscious intensive practice of a certain function.

If you want to develop your brain, you have to choose a function and an area. Building up an area related to juggling might be of little value to your everyday life; working on an area of general functionality would probably be a better use of your time. We have already seen that certain areas of the parietal and frontal lobes seem to be multimodal and, rather than being associated with any one kind of sensory stimulus, are activated during both hearing and vision working memory tasks. Developing a multimodal area would probably be more useful than developing an area that is only related to, say, hearing. These key area also seem to play a part in limiting our capacity to remember information and solve problems.

If we could build up these bottleneck areas through exercise, it would almost certainly be to the benefit of many mental functions. But can we? And if we tried, in what kind of people would the impact of our efforts be most observable? Where do we see the most serious everyday problems with working memory capacity?

9 ■
Does ADHD Exist?

The demands of the information society, with its copious information, simultaneous situations, pace, and distractions, make many of us feel as though we are suffering from some sort of attention deficit. As we have already seen, many of these challenges surrounding us can be traced directly to working memory. Let us, therefore, look more closely at the individuals who have the most serious attention difficulties, and see if these problems can also be linked to working memory.

Lisa is rarely on time for her meetings. She has bought herself a PDA (personal digital assistant), an electronic diary in which she writes down everything she has to do. The PDA then gives a little beep to remind her of what she is to do and when, such as getting ready for her meetings. Yet she often still manages to lose herself in a forest of small details, impulses, and distractions, such as making a call she has suddenly remembered instead of gathering her materials for the meeting. She obeys a sudden impulse to water the plants, which are looking a bit wilted, or goes off with her cup of coffee to the lunchroom, where she forgets what it is she is supposed to do and engages a colleague in conversation about something that has just crossed her mind instead. Consequently, she must scramble to have any hope of making it to the meeting on time. On a number of occasions she has forgotten to pick up her kids from the day care center on time.

The problem, as she puts it, is that the world is moving too quickly. Or is it the thoughts in her head that are moving too quickly? The world seems bursting with details and impressions that she is unable to sort out or bring into any order of priority, and keeping one thought in her head long enough to act on it effectively is beyond her capabilities.

Lisa has taken some steps to deal with this: she has hired an assistant to help keep her on track at work, and she has also begun taking medication to make her feel that the world is moving a little more slowly again—a pair of mental blinkers to keep out some of the torrent of distracting details and impulses that she is unable to fend off by herself.

Most of us suffer from attention deficits to a greater or lesser extent. Our powers of concentration are affected by time of day, lack of sleep, stress, illness, and age. However, there is also a diagnosis that bears this very problem in its name: attention deficit hyperactivity disorder, ADHD for short—which is the diagnosis given to Lisa in the imaginary story above. This condition is defined by eighteen criteria, nine of which are related to attention and nine to impulsivity and hyperactivity. Anyone who meets at least six of the nine attention criteria qualifies for a diagnosis of ADHD, predominantly inattentive type, or attention deficit disorder (ADD), as it is sometimes called. Anyone who also meets at least six of the nine hyperactivity/impulsivity criteria qualifies for a diagnosis of ADHD, combined type.

Let us leave hyperactivity to one side and take a closer look at the attention difficulties. Here are the criteria for attention difficulties from the handbook used by doctors to make their diagnosis:

1. Often fails to give close attention to details or makes careless mistakes in schoolwork, work, or other activities.
2. Often has difficulty sustaining attention in tasks or play activities.
3. Often does not seem to listen when spoken to directly.
4. Often does not follow through on instructions and fails to finish schoolwork, chores, or duties in the workplace.
5. Often has difficulty organizing tasks and activities.
6. Often avoids, dislikes, or is reluctant to engage in tasks that require sustained mental effort.
7. Often loses things necessary for tasks or activities.
8. Is often easily distracted by extraneous stimuli.
9. Is often forgetful in daily activities.

As can be seen from these criteria, the ADHD diagnosis primarily concerns children, although in at least half of affected individuals the symptoms persist into adulthood, especially the attention problems and distractibility; the hyperactivity, on the other hand, often disappears. A number of scientists believe that the type of ADHD that only entails attention difficulties (ADD) should be an independent diagnosis kept separate from other types of ADHD.

ADHD or ADD in adults has received considerable attention in recent years, inspiring a glut of popular science books, Web sites, and online newsgroups. A more lighthearted definition of ADD can be found on the CompuServe ADD Forum, an Internet newsgroup for people with ADD. According to them, "You know you've got ADD when . . . "

- You go to pick up your kids from a friend's, realize that you've missed the house, turn around, and go home—still without the children.
- You notice the burned smell of a pan that's boiled dry. You fill it with water again only to smell that same smell once more thirty minutes later.
- You call a friend to ask her something. By the time she answers (after one ring), you've forgotten the question.
- You go to the bedroom to fetch something, but when you get there you forget what it is you've come in to get.
- You find some food in the microwave in the morning after having been distracted by something the day before and forgotten that you'd put it there.
- The last time you turned up at a meeting punctually was when you forgot to turn your clock back to Standard Time.
- You're introduced to someone and two seconds later forget the person's name.
- You cut short your presentation at work because you've remembered that you've forgotten to turn off your lawn sprinkler. But when you get home, you realize that you forgot to even turn it on.
- You finally remember a job you have to do. When you've assembled the necessary tools, you congratulate yourself—only to discover that you've forgotten that you've already done it.
- You need to take your medicine, and you're there with the pill in one hand and a glass of water in the other. You drink all the water only to notice to your surprise that you're still holding the pill.

■ What Is ADHD?

Delivering a medical diagnosis on the basis of something so arbitrary as a checklist of nine vaguely defined statements might seem absurd. Such objections are justified. There is an element of arbitrariness in using a collection of criteria in this way. On the other hand, however, the same can be said of all psychiatric diagnoses: depression, schizophrenia, and manic-depression are all defined by the fulfillment of a certain number of criteria. One important additional criterion that applies to all psychiatric diagnoses is that the problems are so debilitating that they prevent sufferers from leading a normal life. We all feel a little down now and again, but it is something completely different to be so depressed that you cannot get out of bed in the morning or you attempt suicide. People in this situation need therapy and medical help. To identify who has a degree of crisis that requires help, therapists use a list of criteria. An objective measure this might not be—but it is the best we have at present.

So what about the number of symptoms? Are you healthy if you only have five of the symptoms but sick if you have six? The word *diagnosis* itself calls to mind a black-and-white dichotomy between healthy and sick. When a doctor has to decide whether or not she will prescribe medicine for a patient, she has to categorize the problem: yes or no. However, most scientists see the degree of symptom as being normally distributed among the population. This means that rather than there being a discrete little group of people with attention deficits standing isolated from the healthy masses, there are really only differences of degree. We can compare this to blood pressure, which is also normally distributed. We know that high blood pressure can cause cardiovascular disease and that some people would benefit from medication. To define this group, we need a threshold, above which someone is diagnosed as having hypertension. Terms such as *sick* and *healthy* do not have the same denotations when it comes to normally distributed symptoms.

What, then, are the risks associated with ADHD? Children with ADHD have problems at school. They find it hard to sit still, do their homework, and learn what they need to learn. Their attention problems persist into adulthood, causing similar difficulties in vocational training. They fail at their jobs more often than others and run a higher risk of becoming unemployed. In the long run, there is also a danger of their descending into drug abuse.

There are many interesting questions that can be discussed about ADHD. One concerns heterogeneity, which is to say that the group of people with the ADHD diagnosis have all sorts of symptoms produced by a number of different causes. Most scientists agree that there is no one cause of ADHD—no one gene, no one neurotransmitter, no one brain area. But are there three, fifteen, or five hundred causes?

Those who question the diagnosing of ADHD usually like to blame attention deficits on environmental factors. A diagnosis, especially if the person making it is a doctor, implies that there is a pathology, something biologically amiss with the brain that cannot be fixed, and that there is therefore no point in changing the environment. But do we really have to pit biology and the environment against each other like this? Obviously, ADHD is a problem caused both by an individual's faculties and by the demands of his or her environment. Equally obviously, these faculties reside in the brain—where else? However, the biological nature of the problem does not necessarily preclude our doing anything to address and resolve it, as we saw in the previous chapter on the plasticity of the brain.

In the United States, movements such as Scientology opposes the diagnosing of ADHD and has a literally religious hostility toward medication. Against these tendencies to shut the eyes to the ADHD problem, doctors and scientists are rallying to defend the existence of the diagnosis and the right to treat it with drugs. Moreover, if someone publishes an article on the subject, he or she is usually obliged to follow a list of strict diagnostic criteria. However, if you talk to people on the front line of research, they sometimes say, off the record, that the ADHD diagnosis has had its day and that we have to find more accurate measures. The diagnosis has been important for driving research and is still important for clinical use. However, it is possible that the diagnosis group is too heterogeneous and that the diagnosis is actually hampering research into the causal factors. One possible way forward is to concentrate research on functions instead of diagnoses—for example, to measure different mental functions separately in an attempt to understand how they arose and what can be done about them. This is not to say that the ADHD diagnosis is wrong. What it means is that researchers must be even more accurate if they are to make any headway, in just the same way as in many other fields of science.

To the question "Does ADHD exist?" the answer is: wrong question. There are children and adults with attention deficits. These difficulties are related to differences in biological makeup and are largely hereditary. Comparing ADHD symptoms in identical twins and fraternal twins, we find that as many as 75 percent of the symptoms are congenital, which is high. But the biological nature of a particular phenomenon should not presuppose a simple sick-healthy dichotomy, for, just like blood pressure, there may well be a sliding scale. Nor does this mean that it is permanent or that we should consider it deterministically.

■ The Working Memory Hypothesis

In 1997, Russell Barkley, psychologist and leading ADHD researcher, wrote an article in which he suggested that many of the problems related to ADHD could be attributed to deficiencies in working memory. This was mainly speculation, and there were few studies that had actually measured working memory capacity. However, if we look at the symptoms that define the attention difficulties of ADHD, we usually find many direct ties to working memory and the control of attention.

Criterion 2, "Often has difficulty sustaining attention in tasks or play activities," is effectively the definition of attention control that, as we have seen, overlaps with working memory. Any difficulties a person may have keeping control of her attention could therefore be put down to problems remembering what it is she has to concentrate on.

Criteria 4, 5, and 6 can be attributed to difficulties remembering an instruction or keeping an instruction about what to do next in working memory, something that would clearly make it difficult for a person to organize her work. Criterion 8 is about distractibility, which, as we have seen, is related to working memory capacity. Criterion 9, "Is often forgetful in daily activities," is far too vaguely worded for us to know if it is a matter of long-term memory or something else, although it could be about some form of absentmindedness. Working memory is not everything, and children with ADHD often have other problems that cannot be explained by its limitations. However, working memory failings seem able to explain quite a few of the problems that are usually symptomatic of attention deficits.

Barkley's article sparked a great deal of interest in working memory and ADHD, and there is now a wealth of studies demonstrating working memory deficiencies in children and adults with ADHD. In one study, carried out by our research group at Karolinska Institutet, it was found not only that children with ADHD had a lower working memory capacity but also that this seemed to become progressively worse with age, with the gap between the children with ADHD and the control group widening—an interesting observation that we do not quite know how to explain.

Bearing in mind our discussion in previous chapters on the overlap between the control of attention and working memory, it is perhaps not so surprising to discover that working memory tasks are something that people with ADHD find the hardest to manage. There are also several biological factors tying ADHD to working memory: the areas of the frontal and parietal lobes critical to working memory are, statistically speaking, smaller in people with ADHD, and there are slight abnormalities in the dopamine system, a neurotransmitter network in the brain important to working memory function. For example, it has been found that certain gene variants (alleles) that code for dopamine receptors are more common in people with ADHD. Again, however, there is no absolute dichotomy between people with and without ADHD, a particular gene variant possibly being found in about 40 percent of people with ADHD but in only 20 percent of those without the diagnosis.

■ Pills and Pedagogy

The most important treatment for ADHD is medication with drugs that boost the amount of dopamine available in the synapses. The mechanism of action of these drugs is similar to that of amphetamine, and so they are referred to as central stimulants. The effect of the medicine is remarkable, and it has been called one of the most effective psychopharmaceuticals around. Within only half an hour the children become calmer, less hyperactive, and more focused. Longitudinal evaluations reveal that the drug produces no lasting damage, carries no greater risk of drug dependency, and causes no abnormal brain development. Skeptics, for their part, claim that there are no real control groups for these evaluations and that the studies are based on the much lower drug doses prescribed ten to fifteen years ago. Another point raised by the skeptics is that a recent and extensive study showed that there are no long-term benefits of medication.

One interesting aspect of the medication is that it improves working memory. Swallow a pill and your working memory will improve by some 10 percent (or half a standard deviation of the population, if you have a statistical bent). This is true of people with *and* without ADHD, and it resembles the effects of small doses of amphetamine. The reason seems to be its influence on the dopamine system. Drugs that block dopamine receptors have a detrimental effect on working memory, while drugs that stimulate them have an augmentative effect.

The main alternative to medication is educating parents and teachers to help them better understand and handle the behavior of children with ADHD. One popular training program is called the Community Parent Education Program (COPE) and was designed by Charles Cunningham. Such programs are primarily based on rewarding desired behavior, such as sitting still in the classroom or doing homework, and on managing conflict. They are also more directed toward dealing with children's oppositional behavior. Consequently, their main focus is not on tackling the underlying problems or on analyzing the working memory challenges placed on the children and trying to do something about this aspect of the problem.

If we see difficulties as an imbalance of challenge and skill, children with working memory problems should be treated with measures that reduce the working memory load in the classroom. Ideas such as this are pretty much common knowledge, but they have also been formally collated and applied in Canada through an initiative called TeachADHD. For instance, here is the advice provided on how to modify instructional language:

- Give one direction at a time.
- Make directions clear, short, and specific.
- Repeat the important parts of instructions.
- Provide visual supports for instructions (for example, a checklist of to-do items).

Some modern educational theories say that children should be like little researchers, formulating problems for themselves and seeking the knowledge required to ultimately solve them. This sounds wonderful. However, if you have a poor working memory, the pedagogics of it are a disaster. For someone to organize the material himself, he needs to retain a plan in his working memory. This is much more demanding than when the teacher tells the children what they are to do. Moreover, when many children are engaged in their own projects simultaneously, the level of disturbance in the classroom is much greater. Considered thus, such teaching methodology simply serves to increase in working memory load, and children with difficulties end up lagging even further behind.

Similar advice as that given for teaching children with ADHD is also useful to adults with attention problems. If faced with a large, complex task, some people can have trouble keeping the entire solution plan in their minds. They might therefore find it useful to unpack the plan into a number of small, tangible steps and to write these steps down. Creating a context of structure and organization for themselves is also something with which such people need help. To the easily distracted, a cluttered desk presents a major problem, and their inability to plan a cleanup, with all that such planning entails—when it is to be done, how things are to be organized, sorting out boxes, labels, folders, et cetera—simply leaves their desk in disarray, despite their being the ones most in need of a clean and tidy work surface. It's a vicious circle, in other words.

Kathleen Nadeau, author of the book *ADD in the Workplace*, gives the following tips on how a person with attention deficit can cope with a chaotic office environment:

- Ask for flex time in order to have some less distracting time at work.
- Ask for permission to work at home part of the time.

- Use headphones or a white noise machine to muffle sounds.
- Face your desk away from the flow of traffic.
- Ask to use private offices or conference rooms for periods of time.

In summary, we can say that ADHD or ADD could be seen as an extreme variant of the attention deficit that many of us experience when we are subjected to tougher demands in our work environment and the brain is inundated with more information than our working memories are able to cope with. "Attention deficit trait" is a term coined to describe this very condition. The main message for those encumbered by problems is thus to obtain help with external structures in order to reduce the level of distraction and to relieve the pressure to keep a cognitive hold on plans, both of which strategies entail lightening the load on working memory. But can we not also attack the other front as well? Can we place something in the other pan of the scales and increase our mental capacity?

10 ∎

A Cognitive Gym

Practice makes perfect. Because of the brain's plasticity, practicing a musical instrument causes changes to the cortical areas that control fine motor movement and that perceive notes—and there is nothing to say that we cannot similarly train the areas of the brain the deal with working memory capacity. Despite this, psychologists have customarily treated working memory capacity as something static, an attribute immune to external influence.

To be sure, there are some experiments, largely from the 1970s, in which psychologists tried to improve working memory in their subjects, including children with learning disabilities. In one such study, psychologists tried to teach children strategies for managing working memory tasks. If, for instance, they were required to remember numbers, they might have received an instruction to quietly repeat only the first numbers of the series to themselves and rely on a more passive memory for recalling the last ones. This worked— for numbers. It did nothing, however, to help the children with other mental activities. In other words, there were no secondary effects from learning a particular strategy.

In another heroic study, a college student tried to rote-learn series of numbers being read aloud to him, for one hour a day, three to five days a week, for no less than twenty months. His performance slowly but surely improved, so that by the end of the twenty months he was able to repeat seventy-nine numbers. This does not seem to fit with the idea of the magical number seven. The secret, however, was that the student had worked out strategies for grouping the numbers together and then associating them with information in his long-term memory, in particular his catalogue-like recall of different athletic records, so the sequence 3492 became "3 minutes 49.2 seconds, almost the world record for running a mile," and so forth. After a training session, he could still remember most of the numbers read to him during the day, which shows that what he was drawing on was his long-term memory. When after twenty minutes' training he was tested on a series of letters, he could remember only six. His working memory had not improved.

Learning strategies for recall seems to be of no benefit for any information other than that for which the strategy is being learned. However, rather than learning strategies, the method used in studies of brain plasticity, particularly in primates, was repetitive skill learning. To have an observable effect on the brain, the training had to be of sufficient intensity, in terms of both sessions per day and number of days, as well as repetitive and daily; further, the task had to be of sufficient difficulty, the degree of which is manipulable through automatic methods of adaptation that make the task harder as soon as the performer improves. These principles could also be applicable to working memory training.

What could we theoretically predict about the secondary effects of working memory training? The effects of training are specific to a particular function and the cortical areas it activates. But if there are multimodal working memory areas—areas, in other words, that are activated by different types of working memory task regardless of what it is one has to remember—and if these areas can be built up, there should at least be secondary effects between different types of working memory task. Moreover, we have also seen that the same key areas are activated on the performance of other tasks, such as solving Raven's matrices, so if working memory capacity is improved, secondary effects should be observable in problem-solving activities that use this very faculty.

■ RoboMemo

I became interested in the idea of training working memory toward the end of 1999. If working memory could indeed be developed, it would arguably be of most benefit to those who have the greatest problems with working memory. And it would also probably be in this group where changes would be most salient. As we saw in chapter 9, children with ADHD seem to constitute such a group.

However, the working memory tasks I used in my research were extremely boring, such as remembering the position of circles in a grid. One initial problem was how to make ten-year-old boys and girls, who had trouble sitting still, perform repetitive and monotonous working memory exercises for weeks on end when working memory was the very thing with which they had problems. One solution was to exploit the appeal that computer games have for children and to somehow sprinkle the exercises with a spoonful of sugar that would help the medicine go down. Two game programmers, Jonas Beckeman and David Skoglund, who had designed and programmed a number of play-and-learn games for children between the ages of ten and twelve, helped to give the tasks a more alluring design. As the buttons for the different exercises ended up distributed around the body of a robot, the software came to be dubbed RoboMemo.

In principle, the training program contained the same working memory tasks as I and others before me had used in our research, involving remembering a number of positions presented, or a sequence of digits or letters. The children performed these working memory tasks repeatedly for about forty minutes a day, but always with new combinations of stimuli. As soon as they improved, the level of difficulty was raised, so they were always pushing at the limits of how much information they could remember. To increase motivation even further, we introduced a point system so that the children could compete with themselves and try to beat their own records. We also included at the end, by way of a reward for a hard day's work, a little game in which they could use the points they had earned during the day.

After a number of pilot studies, it was time for the first real test of the training program, for which we used fourteen children with ADHD. There are generally several problems associated with evaluating the effects of training. One of the difficulties with studies in this field is obtaining good comparison groups. If, in order to confirm the efficacy of a treatment on a group of patients, we use a particular task to measure a particular functionality, we will not have taken into account how much of any improvement is attributable to the simple fact that the post-treatment test is the second time they have performed it—what is known as the test-retest effect. Consequently we need a control group, ideally one that performs a task as part of an alternative treatment so that any placebo effect the treatment might have can be ruled out.

For our control version, we opted for a computer program similar to the training one but with easier working memory tasks. In the experimental group, the degree of difficulty of the training program was constantly adapted to the children's abilities, so they alternated between doing experiments in which they were to remember five, six, or seven different digits, while those in the control group only had to remember two. The training effect in the control group was therefore expected to be significantly less, in much the same way as the training effect of lifting half-pound dumbbells is little compared to that obtained by lifting weights at the very limits of your strength.

Children in both groups underwent twenty-five days of training for five weeks and were measured using a variety of tests both before and afterward. When we analyzed the data, we found that those who had undergone the more intensive training not only improved more than the control group on the tasks they had practiced but also showed significant improvements on the working memory tasks that had not formed part of the training program. It seemed, in other words, as if working memory was trainable and that the training had secondary effects.

One drawback of the study was that it used too few subjects. Hardened scientists also pointed out that one study is no study. This is a Catch 22 that most researchers have to put up with and that is encapsulated nicely in this well-known aphorism by psychologist William James: "When a thing is new, people say 'It is not true.' Later, when its truth becomes obvious, they say 'It's not important.' Finally, when its importance cannot be denied, they say 'Anyway, it's not new.'"

Our next task was therefore to substantiate the results in a larger study. This study involved four university hospitals and a total of twenty or so people in different roles. Some fifty children with ADHD sat in front of their computers, either at home or at school, and trained at working memory tasks for five weeks. Using our own specially designed system, the children sent their results via the

Internet to a server at the hospital so that we could monitor them to make sure that they were doing their training properly. After two years of planning, testing, and analyzing, we held in our hands the confirmation we needed of our first study: the working memories of the trained group had improved more than those of the control group. In concrete terms, this meant that the children who had done a certain type of computerized memory task, such as remembering positions in a four-by-four grid and clicking a mouse button, improved at other, noncomputerized types of working memory task too, such as remembering the order in which a psychologist points at wooden blocks glued to a tray in a random formation.

The improvement was 18 percent, and persisted even when we measured the effect three months after training. This means that a subject who could previously hold seven position in his working memory could now hold eight. Achieving a degree of improvement at pointing at blocks might not sound too earth-shattering; nevertheless, what it demonstrates is that working memory can indeed be improved through training. We had shown that the systems are *not* static and that the limits of working memory capacity *can* be stretched.

If we can build up working memory this way, would we not then expect to see an improvement in problem-solving skills too? To investigate this, we turned again to Raven's matrices (see page 142). Even in the first, smaller study we noted that children who trained showed significant improvement on Raven's matrices. This too was corroborated by the second, larger study. The children in the trained group improved by some 10 percent when we retested them, significantly more than the 2 percent improvement registered by the control group.

We also asked the children's parents to assess their everyday behavior using the very same criteria that define ADHD. It turned out that the parents found their children more focused, seemingly confirming the link between ADHD symptoms and working memory that had inspired the study.

Several other research groups have now been able to replicate these findings using our method, including Bradley Gibson and colleagues at the University of Notre Dame, and Christopher Lucas and collaborators at the New York Medical University. They have also been confirmed in a study by Karin Dahlin and Mats Myrberg at the Stockholm Institute of Education, in which children used the training program in the classroom. The method is also being used clinically at various places around Sweden, Germany, Japan, Switzerland, and the United States as an aid to improving working memory, and hence the ability to concentrate, in children with ADHD.

In a large study of the working memory training method, my previous student Helena Westerberg at the Aging Research Center at Karolinska Institutet tested whether working memory could also be improved in healthy elderly people. One hundred people participated in the trial: fifty individuals between twenty and thirty years old and fifty individuals between sixty and seventy years old. Within each age group, participants were randomly assigned to use either the working memory training program we had developed or the placebo version of the program (with easy working memory tasks). All subjects were evaluated on neuropsychological tests before and after training. The results of the tests showed that both young and old participants in the training group improved on working memory tasks that were not part of the training program as well as cognitive tasks such as listening to a continuous stream of numbers and adding the sum of the last two heard digits. The participants were also given a questionnaire about cognitive function in daily life that included questions relating to working memory, such as "Do you often find that you've forgotten what you were going to do when you go from one room to the next?" Perhaps the most surprising result was that although these were healthy subjects, training resulted in a significant decrease in the number of daily cognitive failures and attention problems, and this was true for both the older and younger subjects. This study once again confirms the notion that working memory can be improved by training. Moreover, the study shows that this can be achieved even in older subjects. The effect on daily behavior shows that problems with inattention are actually something that we all have to a greater or lesser extent, and that they are related to working memory.

■ The Effects of Training on Brain Activity

One question that we asked ourselves was whether the effects of working memory training could be seen in changes in brain activity. Can five weeks of cognitive training redraw the map, and if so, at what points? To examine this, we launched a study of young adults without ADHD who were to train their working memories using the same program that we had used in the study of children with ADHD. The reason why we chose to study adults instead of children was that we expected such small changes in brain activity that it would be difficult to measure them if we did not take numerous readings of brain activity over a long period of time. We thought that would be difficult for children to cope with, especially if they found it hard to lie still, which is imperative during an MR scan.

To examine brain activity, we used fMRI to take measurements while the subjects performed first a working memory task and then a control task. All in all, we measured the brain activity of eleven people, eight of whom turned up for examination in the MR scanner on five different days during the training period, giving roughly forty hours of data.

When, after a few months, we started to see the first maps that described which changes were statistically significant, we found that the training had increased the activity of the frontal and parietal lobes. This was interesting for two reasons. First, it demonstrated that intensive, long-term training on a cognitive task can alter brain activity in much the same way that sensory and motor exercise has been shown to do. In earlier research, for instance, scientists had seen that training pitch sensitivity gives rise to an increase in the number of neurons that are involved in the task (see page 98). If the same principle applies to working memory training—that is, the relevant neuron population expands—it would explain the increase in signals that we observed with the MR scanner.

Second, it was interesting to see in which areas we recorded changes. It was not in the visual, auditory, or motor cortices, but in the multimodal "overlap" areas. Moreover, by far the greatest changes were noted in the very same structure, the sulcus intraparietalis, that we have previously associated with the capacity limitations of working memory.

If we look more closely at the scientific literature, we find a whole host of studies that can be interpreted in the same way as ours: namely, that working memory and the control of attentioncan be trained. One of these studies examined a method called "attentional process training," which comprises a number of exercises, such as arranging words in alphabetical order, locating specific targets among distracting stimuli, and classifying words, that subjects are required to perform in the company of a psychologist or an assistant. In one study, the effects of such training were evaluated over a ten-week period in people with different kinds of brain injury. On measuring certain psychological functions, the psychologists found significant improvements in visuospatial working memory (by 7 percent) and on a working memory task that involved adding a series of spoken digits. Interestingly enough, they found no effect on tests measuring stimulus-driven attention.

More recently, in 2008, a research team at the University of Michigan, including Susanne Jaeggi and John Jonides, confirmed the effect of working memory training in a group of young, healthy adults. The participants practiced repetitively on working memory tasks between 8 and 19 days. Practice improved performance not only on working memory tasks, but also on Ravens Progressive Matrices, with the effect being proportional to the number of days of training.

Even though there is still only a handful of studies, the evidence does suggest that working memory can indeed be trained. In this respect, working memory is similar to other motor and sensory skills, the training of which gives rise to changes in the cortical areas that they activate. The areas responsible for keeping information in working memory can be just as plastic as other parts of the brain. We are not talking enormous changes: an 18 percent improvement in working memory and an 8 percent improvement in problem-solving ability. But it does actually seem as if we can stretch the limits of the brain's capacity to handle information. If working memory is so crucial to a number of everyday cognitive activities and can be built up, should we not then constantly be training it? And if such effects were observable, to what activities would this apply?

11 ■

The Everyday Exercising of
Our Mental Muscles

When you wake up in the morning and start to plan your day with its meetings, lunch, travel, and chores, you are doing a mental jigsaw puzzle, the various pieces of which have to be kept in your working memory. You then use your working memory to keep a mental list of the items you need to pack and to remember each one as you look for it.

A little while later, as you read the paper on the subway, you are using your working memory to retain information from the first word of each sentence to the last—a task that is particularly demanding on working memory if you have ended up beside a group of teenagers having an animated discussion about yesterday's soccer game or last Saturday's party. And so we go, using our working memory throughout the day. Should we not therefore be constantly exercising our working memory so that it progressively improves from one day to the next?

The human brain is nature's most complex organ. Although comparing the brain to a muscle is a profanity, at least for a neuroscientist, using a muscular metaphor for working memory is useful for illustrating some principles of training. A muscle such as the biceps, on the front of the upper arm, is used every day when we lift our forearm. It is used when we lift a piece of paper, when we hold our arms over our keyboard, when we pop a tidbit into our mouth, and when we do thousands of other small movements day in and day out. The activation of the muscle prevents it from wasting away, as happens after paralysis. However, the biceps is not strengthened through the act of lifting a sheet of paper. If we want to power it up, we need something heavier. Consulting body-building books, we find that a common recommendation is to select a load that we can barely lift ten times in one go, an exercise that should be repeated three times a session for three sessions a week. This we will have to do systematically for weeks on end before any results can be seen.

Unfortunately, we know considerably less about cerebral exercise than we do about physical exercise. Certain principles, such as taking yourself to the limits of your endurance several days a week for months, can apply in both cases, however. When my research group studied that effects of working memory training in children with ADHD, we compared two groups who differed only in regard to how close to the limits of their capacity they exercised: while the training group carried out working memory tasks containing an information load at the limit of their capacity, the control group carried out tasks requiring little cognitive effort. What we found was that doing simple working memory tasks produced only marginal memory improvements; it was only when the children worked at the limits of their capacity that any real effect could be observed. Moreover, difficulty of task was not the only factor affecting the result: the children had to exercise for at least half an hour a day, five days a week, for five weeks.

Even though different everyday activities vary widely in their cognitive load, how often do we actually exert ourselves to the max? How often do you solve a problem that is almost beyond your capabilities?

■ The Einstein Aging Study

There are studies showing that cognitive ability is affected by daily activities. One such is the Einstein Aging Study, for which Joe Verghese and colleagues at Albert Einstein College of Medicine monitored more than four hundred senior citizens for an average of five years to ascertain how their daily activities affected their cognitive abilities in the long term. Although their particular interest was the development of dementia, they also measured IQ. On several occasions, the subjects were required to take a psychological test and describe in detail their leisure activities, which included reading, writing, crossword solving, board games (chess), participation in discussion groups, playing a musical instrument, playing tennis, golf, swimming, cycling, dancing, gymnastics, bowling, power walking, walking up more than two steps, housework, and child care. They were also asked to state how often they engaged in such activities: daily, several times a week, once a week, once a month, sometimes, or never. The amount of training was converted into a score whereby one point corresponded to one activity once a week. A daily activity therefore gave a score of seven points.

The subjects were followed up about five years later to find out if their leisure activities were having any cognitive effect. To make sure that it was not their original state of health that determined subsequent activity rather than vice versa, adjustments were made for such factors as education, state of health, and initial test results.

What Verghese's team found was that reading, chess, playing a musical instrument, and dancing were all associated with a later relative improvement of cognitive ability and a lower risk of dementia. However, this was the case only if the activities were done several times a week—one game of chess every seven days was not sufficient. If they had a total of eight or more cognitive activity points—if, that is, they did mental exercise at least eight times a week—their risk of developing dementia was halved. The corresponding activity score for physical exercise (cycling, golf, walking, etc.) had, on the other hand, no effect at all on mental health. In other words, while the study shows that everyday mentally demanding activity has an effect, it also reminds us that a certain degree of intensity is required for this to be the case—a principle that applies as much to the mind as it does to the muscles.

Looking through a cognitive lens, we can see that many of the exercises that proved effective in the Einstein Aging Study are the very ones that are known for demanding working memory and control of concentration. Chess was the activity that had the most salient training effect; indeed, thinking several moves ahead is probably one of the most working-memory-loading activities we can do, and this is exactly what we do most of the time during an hour's game. Consequently, the effective time for which we make maximum use of working memory is long. Reading, which the study also showed to be effective, also requires working memory (although the study did not specify whether this correlated with textual complexity, as might be expected). Solving crosswords, which is a popular form of mental gymnastics, had a slight but barely statistically significant positive effect.

Similar results—that cognitive activity helps to ward off dementia—have been produced by Laura Fratiglioni, Bengt Winblad, and colleagues at Karolinska Institutet, who have spent several years evaluating a population of elderly Stockholmers on the island of Kungsholmen. However, their findings are not as negative as those of the Einstein

Aging Study as regards the effects of physical activity, showing as they do that cognitive, physical, and social activity all independently enhance mental health.

So it seems likely that everyday activities can be effective at times. However, if we are to examine the effects of training, we should be more specific. "Use it or lose it" refers to specific functions and areas of the brain. Unfortunately, it was dementia and not working memory that was measured in the Einstein Aging Study, even though those who did not develop dementia performed better on IQ tests. We will therefore be looking at slightly more precise studies of mental training and how they affect mental capacity in a later chapter.

■ Mental Yardsticks

The effects of everyday activities that place demands on working memory probably surround us all the time, although we are not always aware of them. One reason for this is that it is difficult to observe and measure our working memory and powers of concentration for ourselves. If we compare with physical training, it is much more obvious to us that our bodies must be maintained through exercise. We can easily measure the results of our efforts in the gym: we can see how much weight we can lift, time how fast we run our jogging route, and notice that we no longer get out of breath climbing three steps. We can also see with our own eyes how the muscles of strong people are larger, and if we weigh ourselves, we can see how we lose weight when we start to exercise.

Our working memory capacity and powers of concentration are not so immediately obvious; even in environments where working memory is critical—such as in school—they are difficult to observe. Improved performance on an activity is often ascribed to better knowledge and skills: you improve at math because you have committed the rules into long-term memory, , you improve at a musical instrument because you have learnt your scales. The extent to which performance depends on powers of concentration can be difficult to determine; however, with a yardstick of mental activity and concrete feedback on the result of mental training we might one day be able to calculate activity scores in the same way as we now calculate calories or weights at the gym.

Training has been shown by several studies to deliver results if it is done close to the limits of our capacity. What activities place the greatest demands on working memory vary by individual: for a schoolchild, math—especially mental arithmetic—can present the greatest challenge. Reading complex texts in unfamiliar and jargon-heavy fields or long sentences full of difficult lexical items puts large demands on our ability to retain information from the beginning of a sentence while we think about or try to remember the meaning of some difficult piece of terminology. However, our homes are also rife with challenging situations. I myself find it frustratingly difficult to keep in my working memory two lines of a recipe to completion (see Figure 11.1). But I do not spend that many minutes a week following recipes, and so I cannot expect cooking to provide any training.

■ Zen and the Art of Concentrating

If working memory and concentration control are things that we can train, history should give us examples of when this has been done. Let us stick to the theme of attention and training but leap back in time a few centuries. According to *Dialogues of the Zen Masters*, the following scene was acted out some seven hundred years ago:

> One day a man of the people said to Zen Master Ikkyu: "Master, will you please write for me some maxims of

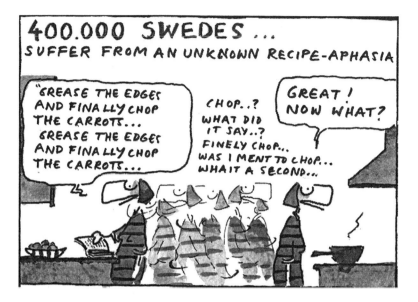

the highest wisdom?" Ikkyu immediately took his brush and wrote the word for "Attention." "Is that all?" asked the man. "Will you not add something more?" Ikkyu then wrote twice running: "Attention. Attention." "Well," remarked the man rather irritably, "I really don't see much depth or subtlety in what you have just written." Then Ikkyu wrote the same word three times running: "Attention. Attention. Attention." Half-angered, the man demanded: "What does that word 'Attention' mean anyway?" And Ikkyu answered gently: "Attention means attention."

The figure of the Buddha with his collected pose and hooded eyes, absorbed in meditation, is the quintessential symbol of concentration. Eastern meditation is often considered the purest form of concentrative activity. But how true is this? Are we talking about powers of concentration in the sense in which experimental psychology and cognitive neuroscience defines it? And does meditation actually improve these skills?

■ *Bompu* Zen

Zen Buddhism is a branch of Buddhism that focuses more on the meditative than the mystical; some even call it more of a philosophy than a religion. Zen evolved as Buddhism migrated from India via China to Japan, where it has been developing since the eighth century.

When practicing Zen, you sit with your eyes half shut, trying to concentrate on your posture and breathing; there is no mantra or visualization of your inner light, and usually you count breaths, a number for every breath, until you get to ten, at which point you start again. The function of this counting is to alert you to when your thoughts start to wander—if you lose count or notice that you have just counted breath number sixteen, you realize that you have lost concentration and have to reset your counter to one. Many people believe that meditation is very much like concentration training.

The Japanese Zen master Yasutani Roshi (1885–1973) grouped Zen Buddhist practice into five types, of which the first, *bompu* Zen, is devoid of any specific philosophical or religious content:

> Through the practice of *bompu* Zen you learn to concentrate and control your mind. It never occurs to most people to try to control their minds, and unfortunately this basic training is left out of contemporary education, not being part of what is called acquisition of knowledge. Yet, without it what we learn is difficult to retain because we learn it improperly, wasting much energy in the process. Indeed, we are virtually

crippled unless we know how to restrain our thoughts and concentrate our mind.

The concepts of "controlling" and "concentrating" the mind seem very close to the notion of control of attention. It is also interesting to read how critical he believes this skill to be to so many mental activities and how much he regrets that, despite its trainability, it is ignored in schools—as are working memory and the powers of concentration. What is needed is greater awareness of the very existence of "control of attention" followed by systematic training to strengthen them.

Science and Meditation

The new millennium has brought a reawakened interest among neuroscientists in questions that were previously considered too "fluffy" to touch. It is now acceptable to delve into consciousness and the brain activity associated with it. Meditation too has seen something of a renaissance, a sign of which was the invitation to the Dalai Lama to speak at the 2005 Conference of the Society for Neuroscience, which with over twenty thousand attendees is the largest congress in the field. The Dalai Lama talked about his interest in science and urged scientists to devote more of their work to empathy. He has also professed himself willing to abandon any Buddhist tenet that can be disproven by science—a promise that would seem quite safe to make, given that many Buddhist beliefs, such as reincarnation, are virtually impossible to invalidate.

At a number of U.S. centers, including the University of California at Davis, Princeton, and Harvard, research is being conducted into meditation. At one conference of neuroscientists and Buddhists, Nancy Kanwisher, a leading cognitive neuroscientist, noted, "Training the attention has barely been touched by cognitive neuroscience."

Only a few studies have been published on the topic. A search of several medical and psychological databases for scientific publications gives countless references to how the relaxing effect of meditation can be used to alleviate anxiety, lumbar pain, stress, headaches, and cocaine abuse, and how it affects the immune system, skin conductance, and melatonin secretion—but there are still few hard facts on its role in improving concentration.

One study of the brain and meditation was led by Richard Davidson at the University of Wisconsin, who is, incidentally, a Buddhist and a personal friend of the Dalai Lama. The study, which used electroencephalography (EEG) to measure the electrical currents generated by neuronal activity, involved eight Tibetan Buddhist monks with between ten thousand and fifty thousand hours' experience of meditation, and ten college students, who were all asked to meditate on the theme of "unconditional love" while being monitored.

The monks achieved a stronger signal of the higher (gamma) frequencies, which are thought to be important for binding the activity of different parts of the neocortex. However, it is not clear just how we are to interpret the differences observed between the monks and the students.

An fMRI study of the brain activity of Buddhist monks was published in 2007 by Julie Brefczynski-Lewis and Richard Davidson. Once inside the MR scanner, the monks were asked to concentrate on a dot on a screen in front of them. What they found was that the monks evinced higher brain activity than a control group in the same areas (in part) of the frontal lobe and the sulcus intraparietalis that have already been associated with the control of concentration and where we have also found an increase in activity after working memory exercises. It would seem that here too, albeit indirectly, are links between the control of concentration and the attention that is developed through meditation.

Another study from 2007 comparing thirteen Zen practitioners and thirteen controls found that the meditators had superior performance on a computerized test of controlled attention and that the normal age-related decline in gray matter volume and reaction time was much less pronounced.

There is such a wealth of activities that fall under the category of meditation that it is impossible to make any general claim about attention and meditation. Even what one would think is a rather well-defined form of meditation—Rinzai-school Zen Buddhist meditation—apparently contains at least five different types, each with its own purpose. However, apart from the practice offering more spiritual rewards, much of this meditation, or *bompu* Zen, seems devoted to the control of attention. The study conducted by Brefczynski-Lewis and Davidson also suggests that the cerebral effects of a certain type of meditation can correlate with the systems that we know are involved in the control of concentration. Sometimes attention is just attention.

■ Current and Future Challenges

But let us return to the present and, above all, to how changes in our environment influence the mental challenges we face. Many situations that place significant demands on working memory are associated with new technology, such as learning how to work a new gadget or computer program. Let us say that you are using a word processing program and want to hyphenate your text. Since you have no idea how to do this, you activate the help function. Here you find the following information: "1. On the *Tools* menu, point to *Language*, and then click *Hyphenation*. 2. Select the *Automatically hyphenate document* check box. 3. In the *Hyphenation zone box*, enter the amount of space to leave between the end of the last word in a line and the right margin." Anyone who manages to keep this instruction in working memory deserves applause.

Changes in society, with its growing volume of complex texts and instructions, its ever more mind-boggling technology, its simultaneous situations, and its never-ending stream of latest-version software, should put increasing pressure on our working memories in our everyday lives. The remainder of this book will look beyond the laboratory to possible examples of training results in different contexts. One activity that has grown particularly popular in recent years is playing computer games. What effect do these things have? Do they do a disservice to children's powers of concentration, as some people fear, or actually improve them?

12 ∎

Computer Games

Jennifer Grinnell, who lives in Michigan, has quit her old job at a furniture company and now devotes herself full-time to the virtual world of Second Life. Second Life is a *massively multiplayer online game* (MMOG), in which users hook up to the Internet to enter an imaginary 3-D environment that they can navigate, buying buildings and land and creating their own virtual objects, such as furniture and clothes, as well as their own character (called an *avatar*).

Jennifer's specialty is designing clothes and appearances that other players can then buy and use for their avatars. After one month in Second Life, she was earning more on the game than she was in her old job at the furniture company. After three months, she quit her day job to devote herself full-time to the game, in a world that she shares with millions of other users. Some people play just for the experience, others to earn money. The community that has evolved has become the subject of study for university economics students. There are also sociological projects going on around Second Life, such as investigating whether disabled children can be helped to integrate into the virtual world in a way that would be impossible in the real world.

Jennifer Grinnell is an extreme example of how computer games create alternative worlds into which more and more people are devoting more and more time. Second Life is also an example of the breadth of digital entertainment that is out there enticing us. If we are going to look for activities in our everyday lives that can affect our powers of concentration, it is not chess or crosswords that we should turn to but computer games. All ages play computer games, but they are still largely the domain of children and teenagers. Computer game playing has evolved from being a pastime for a minority of computer enthusiasts to a major leisure time activity. The vast amount of time that many children dedicate to playing gives the activity the potential to affect the brain and the cognition. The question is how.

Many parents are worried about what computer games might be doing to their children. There are three main fears: that the violence depicted in the games will make them more aggressive, that the lack of exercise will make them fat, and that the nature of the medium will induce concentration problems and ADHD-like symptoms. The debate on violence in computer games resembles the one that has raged for decades on violence in films, and although the question is worth taking seriously, it belongs to another forum. The issue of how the lack of exercise affects children is also important, but I will gladly hand that over to dietitians and those who decide how much PE should be in the school curriculum. Let us focus instead on if and how playing computer games affects our powers of concentration.

■ Scares

This is what the British newspaper *The Observer* wrote in 2001:

> Computer Games Stunt Teen Brains
> Hi-tech maps of the mind show that computer games
> are damaging brain development and could lead to
> children being unable to control violent behaviour
>
> Computer games are creating a dumbed-down
> generation of children far more disposed to violence than
> their parents, according to a controversial new study. The
> tendency to lose control is not due to children absorbing
> the aggression involved in the computer game itself, as
> previous researchers have suggested, but rather to the
> damage done by stunting the developing mind.

The study referred to was carried out by Ryuta Kawashima, a Japanese neuroscientist from Tohoku University (who never published the story, but instead later collaborated with Nintendo to create the Brain Age software).

Kawashima and his team measured the blood flow in the brains of children in three different situations: while playing computer games, while resting, and while doing repetitive arithmetical exercises (adding single-digit numbers). The games had a sports theme and, designed for a Nintendo Game Boy (a small handheld console particularly popular with young children), were relatively basic.

They found that whereas the games only really activated the visual and motor cortices, the arithmetical exercises activated the frontal lobes. It is also possible that the differences in activity patterns are related to the games' heavy demands on stimulus-driven attention, rewarding speed of stimulus response but requiring little working memory. The arithmetical exercises, however, demand a great deal from working memory and therefore activate the frontal lobes. This said, the only conclusion we can draw from the study is that sports computer games do not activate the frontal lobes.

We could, of course, conclude that it is unlikely that sports computer games enhance frontal lobe function, although this is a characteristic that such games probably share with many other activities, perhaps even real sports too. There is nothing in the study to suggest that the activity registered during the games is in any way lasting or that playing computer games leads to violent behavior. Further, they did not measure behavioral changes and used no test of attention or working memory. The contrast between the study's actual results and the *Observer*'s interpretation is striking, and shows how easily disinformation is spread by the media.

■ The Benefits of Computer Games

A number of cross-sectional studies comparing young people who devote much of their time playing computer games with young people who do not have shown that children who play a lot of computer games perform worse at school; others, contradicting this, have found that those who play least are at the greatest disadvantage. One problem with this kind of study is that it is sometimes very difficult for the scientists to control for all background factors and to ensure that the children who play a lot do not differ from the control group in other respects than just playing habits; further, they have not been measuring the subjects' powers of concentration or working memory. Because of this, the conclusions ought to be confirmed through experimental studies, in which people are randomly assigned to two different groups, one of which gets to play computer games, and evaluated both before and afterward.

One such experimental study assessed the effects of Tetris, a game in which variously shaped polygons descend slowly from the upper edge of the screen's playing field. As they fall, players can rotate and translate them laterally to make them fit with the spaces left by the shapes accumulating beneath them. It turned out that eleven days of Tetris playing left the subjects better able than the controls to solve visuospatial problems, such as piecing together shapes into a pattern, a task not unlike that used in IQ testing to evaluate spatial skills.

One of the few studies that has closely measured the effects of action games on attention is described by Shawn Green and Daphne Bavelier of the University of Rochester. In the first part of the study, Green and Bavelier compared frequent players of computer games with people who played them rarely or never. The groups were comparable in all other respects such as age, sex, and educational background. The team compared the groups' performances on several tasks measuring visual perception. In one test, they flashed a number of objects onto a screen and then asked the subjects to say how many items they had seen. This is usually quite easy to do with three objects, but when faced with four, the control group gave incorrect responses roughly 10 percent of the time. The experimental group was much better at this task than the controls, reaching up to six objects before displaying the same kind of failure rate.

In another test, they measured speed of attention. The subjects were shown a series of letters on a screen one at a time, so quickly that they barely had time to register them. Their task was to press a button as soon as they saw the target, which was the letter A. It is a well-known psychological effect that when we register a target, our ability to identify new targets coming in close succession is slightly impaired by a split-second "attentional blink." In the computer playing group, this blink was shorter than it was in the control group, allowing them to identify new targets after the first with greater speed.

To make sure that the group of computer game players did not differ in other respects (age, sex, and educational background) from the control group, and that there was therefore no hidden explanation for the differences observed between the groups, the study was complemented with a further experiment. This second study randomly allocated nonplayers only to two groups, one of which played the action game Medal of Honor and the other—the control group—Tetris. After one hour's play a day for ten days, the subjects were evaluated with the same tests used in the first part of the study. Again, improvements were observed in the experimental group, corroborating the results of the first part of the study.

Whether the tests on which the participants improved measure perceptual ability, perceptual speed, or (as the authors interpret it) stimulus-driven attention is a moot point. What is undeniable is that computer games improve certain functions. The second part of the experiment, in which a comparison was made with Tetris, is also interesting in that it shows how specific the effects of different computer games are. It is therefore futile to talk about computer games as a homogenous group without specifying the genre and looking more closely at the skills they develop. Action games are the ones to have received most media attention, but the top-selling game is The Sims, in which players have to optimize their virtual characters' social life and well-being, furnish their house, and make sure that they turn up at work on time.

The National Institute of Public Health in Sweden has recently published a report systematically reviewing thirty published studies on the effects of computer games. It found a total of six studies that all demonstrated an enhancement of spatial skills and reaction times. No studies showed any deleterious effect on attention.

■ Computer Games and the Future

There is thus no evidence that computer games impair people's attention or induce ADHD in young players. New findings are constantly being published, so it is impossible to make any categorical pronouncement on the matter, but one reason to be skeptical about any link between concentration problems and computer games is that there is, as yet, no mechanism to explain how any such connection would come about. We would, for instance, need studies establishing a general principle that strengthening stimulus-driven attention weakens controlled attention, and there are none supporting this. When psychologists measure stimulus-driven and controlled attention in a large population, they find that they are statistically unrelated. Your math skills do not suffer when you play soccer or study French.

There is, of course, a certain give-and-take in everything you do since there are only twenty-four hours in the day, so if a child spends a lot of time playing computer games, it leaves little time for math homework—although this perhaps applies even more to watching TV, which is a more passive pastime and one that deprives us of the opportunity to develop our working memories by spending time on something more cognitively demanding. It is not the quick-fire editing or the overabundance of information in the programs themselves that has this negative effect; indeed, the same outcome of mental sedentariness would be caused by other activities that do not train working memory. In the Einstein Aging Study, a weak (nonsignificant) negative effect was observed in those who spent a lot of time cycling.

But even if playing computer games was a waste of time, it is also possible, as the Tetris study and Green and Bavelier show, that it produces certain enhancements, such as of visuospatial and perceptual skills. Each computer game is different depending on the skills it rewards.

There are a number of programs of the "play and learn" kind, which teach children things such as spelling, foreign languages, or math through games; most of these involve either the drilled consignment of knowledge to long-term memory or the practice of a specific skill. Another type of program that has started to appear on the Internet has been developed to train certain fundamental cognitive functions, including working memory and attention. Superficially, these programs are more like neuropsychological tests than training programs, and they contain a range of exercises such as recalling numbers or testing reaction times. I concede that many of these programs might be beneficial, but they also contain exercises that are probably devoid of all function. Insofar as they have not been properly evaluated, it is impossible for us to know what is effective and what is a waste of time. For there to be any effect, we would need not only to do the right kinds of exercise but also to do them in a way that brings about lasting change, which is to say at the right level of difficulty and with sufficient intensity for a sufficient length of time. Logging on to the Internet and playing a few games once a week is unlikely to have any enduring effect.

Seriousgames.org is an initiative that brings together different projects designed to use gaming technology to improve performance in areas of health care and leadership, with titles such as Laser Surgeon: The Microscopic Mission, Life and Death II, and SimHealth. One interesting game in this field has been produced by Applied Cognitive Engineering, a company that has settled into the rather narrow niche of improving the cognitive skills of basketball players. The training program, called Intelligym, is designed to improve what they call *game intelligence*, which comprises a battery of basic skills such as attention, decision making, and spatial perception. The software was originally developed to improve the performance of Israeli fighter pilots; it is now marketed, in a modified version, to professional basketball teams. The program is claimed to be able to boost a team's performance by 25 percent, although there are no controlled studies to show that it actually works (or if there are, they constitute military secrets and are in the safe custody of the Israeli army).

Perhaps one day we will see games that exploit the knowledge about training effects that we are now starting to obtain, and combine the allure of the adventure and action genres with play that enhances problem solving and working memory. One sign that the trend is coming is the entrance of Nintendo into the arena with the launch of Brain Age: Train Your Brain, a game designed to train users' brains by requiring them to do certain tasks, such as solving fairly simple mathematical problems. The game has been developed for their latest handheld console, but is aimed mainly at adults wanting to keep their brains in trim. At the end of a round, the estimation of the brain's age is updated: if you have done well, your brain age decreases; if you have done poorly, you watch your brain take another step toward the dark abyss of dementia. The game is selling in the millions.

Personally, I feel that the tasks presented in the game are too rudimentary to have any real training effect. Not surprisingly, there is also no study to show that the game has any impact whatsoever on the brain in general or a specific cognitive function in particular. Moreover, the games are too boring for users to want to stick with them long enough to have any effect (assuming, that is, that they are capable of having an effect). However, the game itself and the fact that it has been developed by Nintendo suggest the start of a trend, and new games in the same genre are already filling the shelves.

A more scientific approach is taken by the company Posit Science, which has Michael Merzenich as its lead scientist. A large study found some effect of their brain training program, although it did not survive a direct comparison with the control group. The company Lumosity has marketed cognitive training on-line. There is as yet (2008) no published studies of this method, but according to the company "white paper" there is some effect on visual perception but the effect for improvement of working memory is extremely small.

A little over a century ago, children were being told to go out and play or help in the garden instead of doing something as unnatural as lying down for hours on end with their nose in a book. Reading was thought to addle their brains, make them weak, and ruin their eyes. As it turned out, reading offered excellent preparation for the dawning information society. Perhaps playing computer games provides a similar grounding for the information intensive and digitalized future that awaits us.

So what are our working memories like, on average? What about the aggregate effect of the environmental changes we can see taking place around us? Do we generally have worse powers of concentration owing to the continual distractions around us, and are we all generally destined to develop attention deficit trait? Or do the greater demands and challenges of our society, including perhaps the games we play, mean that we are forever training our cognitive faculties?

13 ■
The Flynn Effect

As we have already discussed, New Zealand professor James Flynn demonstrated how IQ performance improved throughout the 1900s—and what improvements they were. If the average performance in 1932 was 100, by 1990 it was 120. A person who scored an average 100 in 1990 would therefore be able to count herself among the top 15 percent if she went back in time to 1932. According to some, it also seems as if the curve is steepening. What was once an average IQ increase of 0.31 IQ point per year in the 1950s, 1960s, and 1970s had risen to 0.36 IQ point per year by the 1990s. This result is surprising, since it was previously thought that intelligence was a constant. But an ever-expanding file of studies suggests that this is not the case.

Given that many people cock their revolvers as soon as they hear the word *intelligence*, maybe it would be a good idea at this point to say a few words about what scientists usually mean by the term. When we give a large number of psychological tests to a large number of people, we find that performance on the tests is positively correlated. This means that those who perform above average on one test usually perform above average on other tests too, suggesting the presence of a factor affecting performance on all tests. This hypothetical factor can be found using statistical methods and has been given the designation g, for "general factor." *IQ* stands for "intelligence quotient," the quotient obtained by dividing measured mental age by actual age and multiplying by 100.

The number of factors and what they represent was the topic of much psychological debate in the 1900s. One of the most influential theories was posited by American psychologists Raymond Cattell and John Horn, who argued that two of the most important factors are *crystallized* and *fluid* intelligence. Crystallized intelligence (gC) accounts for performance on tasks dealing with vocabulary and general knowledge; fluid intelligence (gF), on the other hand, explains why people differ in performance on nonverbal problem-solving and reasoning tasks that are independent of general knowledge.

Further, Swedish researcher Jan-Eric Gustafsson has shown that the factor most related to g is gF, with which Raven's matrices are a closely correlated task (see Figure 13.1). By definition, then, fluid general intelligence is something that can only be measured with a large battery of tests. However, gF correlates so highly with performance on Raven's matrices that sometimes psychologists feel that they need only measure performance on these tasks in order to make a somewhat casual pronouncement about gF. And this is where working memory comes in too. As we have seen in an earlier chapter, performance on working memory tests and performance on Raven's matrices are also highly correlated, prompting many to argue that working memory capacity is the most critical underlying gF determiner.

■ Developing Your IQ

If environmental conditions influence gF, it should also be trainable, so let us look more closely to see if there are any studies corroborating this. One of the best and largest training studies ever performed was Project Intelligence, which was carried out in the poorer parts of the city of Barquisimeto in central Venezuela in the early 1980s. The project was initiated by the national government but was conducted with researchers from Harvard. A program was drawn up by teachers and scientists to train thirteen- and fourteen-year-old schoolchildren in "observation skills and classification, deductive or inductive reasoning, critical use of language, problem solving, inventiveness and decision-taking." The experimental group comprised 463 pupils, who took special classes for a full academic year, and the control group 432 pupils, who received the normal curriculum. A large number of tests were done before and after the study period to measure general intellectual functions, such as problem solving and logical reasoning.

The results were very positive for most of the tests. The group that had received the special training improved their mean performance by roughly 10 percent. Put a little crassly, this means that, accounting for the normal yearly progress of the control group, the experimental group increased its IQ by 10 percent. It also seemed as if all pupils improved to the same extent irrespective of age, sex, and initial test results, implying that the special education was not only of benefit to those who scored low on the pre-study test.

Another example of the effects of training is a study showing how Israeli underachievers could improve their IQs by taking a problem-solving course known as *instrumental enrichment*. Interestingly enough, the differences between the experimental group and the control group did not disappear once the training had come to an end; in fact, the effects of the training escalated from year to year. This can be interpreted as the result of a positive feedback loop: improved abilities give more intellectual stimulation, which in turn fuels the abilities. A child who improves his problem-solving skills will find it easier to do his math homework. This will encourage him to spend more time with math, which in turn will bring about an even greater improvement of his problem-solving skills. This positive feedback effect is something that has previously been observed in studies of children with reading difficulties. Once they have undergone intensive training programs, children become more effective readers; they consequently spend more time reading every day, which in turn hones their reading skills even more.

One series of studies was carried out by the Yugoslavian psychologist Radivoy Kvashchev. Although he only published his results in Serbo-Croatian, one of his students made his results available in English. In one of his larger studies, 296 students were trained in "creative problem solving" for three to four hours a week for three years. Compared with a control group, these students showed an improvement of 5.7 IQ points, which is roughly the same in percentage. On a follow-up a year after their training program had finished, he found that this difference had risen to 7.8 points—again, a higher score on a subsequent measure that could be the result of positive feedback.

In a German training study led by Karl Klauer, seven-year-olds were given training in "inductive reasoning," which involves the ability to recognize patterns and then formulating and applying a rule, in much the same way as when solving a Raven's matrix. The tasks were of the "odd man out" kind, in which the subject has to work out which three of a group of four objects belong together and, accordingly, which one has to be discarded. The children were taught in small groups and were given two lessons a day for five weeks. Compared with a passive control group, they found that the experimental group improved on Raven's matrices, an effect that persisted for another six months.

To the string of studies that have been shown to improve fluid intelligence we can also add the results obtained by my own team and the study of working memory training by Susan Jaeggi and collegues. When children with ADHD trained their working memories, we noted an 8 percent improvement in performance on Raven's matrices (after having subtracted that recorded in the control group). The degree of magnitude of this improvement is also the same as that obtained in Project Intelligence as well as by Kvashchev and Klauer.

It stands to reason that problem-solving abilities should improve with working memory, bearing in mind the known link between these two phenomena. Perhaps it is even the case that working memory is the very part of our intellectual faculties that is developable and that this is the core of the various training studies. The ability to improve working memory through training might well be the key to understanding the entire Flynn effect.

■ Everything Bad Is Good for You

Studies of how training and specially designed teaching improve IQ thus provide grist for the mill of those who claim that IQ is not just inherited. Intelligence is not an absolute cognitive tool with which we are equipped from birth. If training can be shown to influence IQ, we should also see effects from our psychological environment in general. In *The Rising Curve*, published in 1988, an assortment of leading psychologists discuss how the Flynn effect could be attributed to our environment. In an article entitled "The Cultural Evolution of IQ," Patricia Green argues it was the heavier information flow and the greater complexity of society that had the greatest effect on IQ during the last decades of the twentieth century.

The same point, though much expanded upon, was made by author Steven Johnson in *Everything Bad Is Good for You*. His main thesis is that mass culture has, on average over the past thirty years, become increasingly complex and mentally challenging rather than simpler and dumbed-down, and that for some reason the media gear themselves more toward those who demand more rather than to the lowest common denominator. He also suggests that this greater complexity is one of the causes of the Flynn effect.

When it comes to TV and film, this greater complexity resides partly in the way they require us to keep tabs on several parallel plotlines. If we were to trace the dramatic trajectory of *Starsky and Hutch*, a TV cop show from the 1970s, we would end up with a straight line: each episode involved the same two lead characters and had one story line, excepting an introduction and an ending. Similarly charting an episode of *Seinfeld* or *The Sopranos* twenty years later would reveal a much more complex tissue of five or ten interwoven thematic threads.

Another factor that has increased narrative complexity is the partial withholding of context and information, which forces viewers to work out the circumstances or conversational references for themselves. Instead of just sitting and thinking, "I wonder what'll happen at the end," they spend much of the time thinking, "I wonder what's happening now"—a continual process of problem solving, in other words. Often, the chronological sequence of contemporary film plots is so fragmented that the viewers are left with little choice but to constantly fit the pieces together if they are to work out how what they are currently seeing relates to what they have seen thus far. This is a particularly demanding exercise.

Johnson also writes at some length about computer games as an example of life's increasing complexity. That a game such as Grand Theft Auto (in which players steal cars and joyride through a virtual city in order to perform tasks

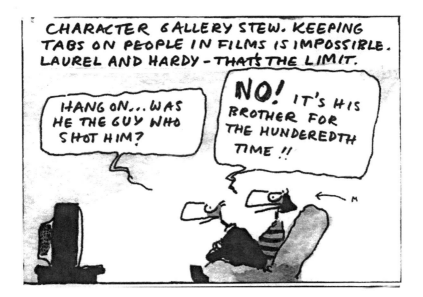

FIGURE 13-1
© Jan Berglin.

of varying degrees of nefariousness), with its two-hundred-
page manual, is more complex than Pac-Man is something
on which most of us would agree. It can be harder, though,
to put our fingers exactly on where this complexity resides.
Johnson suggests that is has two components: *probing* and
telescoping. The probing is a result of the lack of clarity in the
rules, which forces the player to work out for herself what
she has to do and how she has to do it. This she does by probing, generating hypotheses on how the game works and
repeatedly testing these hypotheses by probing even more.

Telescoping involves working through problems comprising a hierarchy of goals and subgoals. The Legend of
Zelda: The Wind Waker is a Japanese adventure game designed originally for the handheld Game Boy but which
went on to be adapted for more powerful consoles. The basic game plot involves a young boy from a small island
who goes out into the big wide world to save a kidnapped

girl. Just like in Grand Theft Auto, the plot is hardly high literature. Johnson's point is that cognitive challenges can exist even in a rather trivial narrative context. To illustrate, one mission from Zelda is built up as follows:

> You have to meet a prince to give him a letter.
> To do that, you have to climb a mountain.
> To do that, you have to make your way to the other side of a gorge.
> To do that, you have to fill the gorge with water so that you can swim across.
> To do that, you have to use a bomb to blow up the boulder blocking a spring.
> To do that, you have to grow a bomb plant.
> To do that, you have to collect water in a bottle you were given by the girl.

Telescoping thus consists of organizing a sequence of sub-goals while keeping them alive in the mind.

Green and Johnson both probably have a point. But neither of them manages to find a precise measure for what it is they mean by complexity. And because they cannot measure their complexity, they cannot show that the complexity has actually increased, and thus lack any data to demonstrate the effects of training.

However, some of what Johnson calls complexity probably has something to do with working memory load. His definition of telescoping, for instance, is to retain a number of subgoals in the head, in exactly the same way as in working memory tasks. If we read "working memory load" instead of "complexity," we could reconcile his ideas with studies that demonstrate the effects of working memory training, the results of the Einstein Aging Study, and the improvement in problem-solving skills seen in Project Intelligence, the Israeli study, and the work of Klauer and Kvashchev. If we assume that all these phenomena are related and that it is the working memory effect that lies behind the Flynn effect, the implications are revolutionary. Maybe we live in a society in which games, media, and information technology are putting an ever-increasing load on our working memory. This, in turn, is improving the average working memory and problem-solving skills of the population at large, which in turn ups the load and the complexity. Is the human norm being raised?

14 ■
Neurocognitive Enhancement

So the Flynn effect reflects how general intelligence is progressively increasing with time. Will this trend continue, with the growing demands of our environment matched by our equally expanding capacity? Will scientists be able to use our knowledge of the brain to boost its capacity further?

In the introduction to this book, I cited an article by some neuroscientists who claimed that "humanity's ability to alter its own brain function might well shape history as powerfully as the development of metallurgy in the Iron Age." The authors aimed to identify a trend of *neurocognitive enhancement* and to provoke discussion on a number of related issues. Neurocognitive enhancement denotes the use of existing and potential techniques, such as brain-computer interaction, neurosurgery, and psychopharmacology, to exploit the brain's capacity for change.

The first problem addressed by the authors is what happens when an agent, such as a medication, changes from being a means of curing people with some impaired function to a tool for boosting the faculties of the healthy.

The second problem raised by the article is more philosophical. Improving cognitive function is not just like tweaking a car engine. Psychoactive substances can also affect the personality. The danger, they argue, is that we become different people with such drugs in our body compared to who we are without them, which can induce psychological problems about identity and raise philosophical issues about responsibility.

■ Mental Doping

One class of drug that is often discussed is the central stimulant, which has already been described in the chapter on ADHD. What was first thought a particular effect on the mental capacity of people with concentration problems later turned out to be a general effect. In one of the first studies on this, led by Judith Rapoport at the National Institute of Mental Health, a group of nonhyperactive boys between the ages of seven and twelve with above-average cognitive skills were given either a placebo or a low dose of amphetamine usually given to children with ADHD, and then tested. What they found was that the cognitive skills of the boys in the amphetamine group also improved. They sat more still but also asked fewer questions.

More recent studies have demonstrated similar effects for methylphenidate (Ritalin). If we measure the effects of amphetamine or methylphenidate with psychological tests, we find that they increase arousal, speed up reaction times, improve working memory capacity by about 10 percent, and significantly mitigate symptoms of hyperactivity and concentration deficit. The fact that methylphenidate also works in people without ADHD is not particularly surprising, given that people do not simply fall into two convenient groups, one with and one without concentration problems. Instead, there is a very fluid boundary between different degrees of concentration ability. Knowledge of the general effects of methylphenidate has also spread, especially to university students, who have started to use the drug when studying for exams. Some reports also claim that 16 to 18 percent of university students in the United States use stimulants to improve their study performance. A 2008 survey by the scientific journal *Nature* revealed that about 20 percent of the responants took drugs for cognitive enhancement. In Japan, the nonprescription use of Ritalin was considered so widespread that the authorities eventually decided to impose a total ban on the drug.

It is, then, largely the increasingly widespread use of the drug by people who have not been diagnosed with ADHD that is raising fears. Can its growing popularity make those who do not take it feel compelled to do so? Might teachers recommend that certain students take it to enable them to keep up with their classmates? Will employees be expected to take their morning pill to remain in the promotion machine or to even keep their jobs?

Ritalin was the first of these drugs on the market and is the most widespread. However, there is much to suggest that we will see more of other cognition-enhancing drugs in the future. Forty or so other substances are being developed out of our increasingly detailed knowledge of the cellular processes involved in the encoding of long-term memory. One class of substances, known as ampakine drugs, facilitates this encoding process; another drug, MEM1414, developed by a company with the science-fiction-like name of Memory Pharmaceuticals (cofounded by Nobel laureate Eric Kandel), will make it easier to strengthen the connections between neurons, and with them long-term memory. Anyone who might be scared by the idea that each and every insignificant detail will be imprinted forever in their memories if they start to use these substances can relax, as other substances for erasing long-term memories are also under development—presumably for use with conditions such as post-traumatic stress syndrome.

Knowledge of the memory's cell biology has also led to the successful genetic modification of mice to make them better at performing memory tests. What next? In sports, much concern has been expressed about gene doping. Can we imagine similar doping for the improvement of cognitive function? Human-computer interaction has fascinated science fiction writers for decades. In 2006, scientists demonstrated how they could feed the brain signals of a paralyzed person into a computer and use them to operate a mechanical arm. If we can learn the principles by which neurons can be directly integrated with computers, our future possibilities will be enormous. Maybe we will be able to use computers as an extra plug-in memory for our brains and upgrade our working memory every other year?

■ Our Daily Drugs

The idea of using artificial means to improve the brain is interesting but actually not new. It is only the substances that are new. Caffeine is a substance that is very similar in effect to amphetamine and one that we have been self-administering for centuries. Caffeine allows us to conquer fatigue when we have been sleeping badly and to work more hours of the day than we otherwise would. We can therefore feel justified in claiming that coffee changes the standard for what is an acceptable level of tiredness. Yet we have adapted to this—so is there any moral dilemma here? Do we feel forced by our boss to drink coffee? Does coffee change our personalities?

Other trends we are warned of include the use of drugs developed to treat diseases or deficiencies to boost the performance of healthy people. This trend is also now with us. One such example is the use of estrogen to offset the completely natural hormonal decline that takes place in women as they get older. We find similarly normal age-related trends in the brain. The concentration of dopamine receptors, for instance, drops steadily from the age of twenty-five at an estimated rate of about 8 percent a decade. The loss of dopamine receptors might account for the progressive deterioration of working memory with age. Ritalin affects the availability of dopamine, so if we allow the replacement of estrogen, why should we not also allow the replacement of dopamine? My guess is that in fifteen years' time, middle-aged people will be regularly imbibing a cocktail of substances designed to counteract the completely natural decline in various neurotransmitters in the brain, in exactly the same way as some women today take estrogen.

Many of the future trends about which the authors talk are already here. Our carefree use of other drugs might mean that we gradually become inured to the use of other drugs and techniques. What will prove decisive in shaping developments in this respect might not be any ethical stance but simply the demonstrated efficacy of the drugs and their possible long- or short-term side effects.

This is no small practical aspect but a crucial and complex matter. I would love to take a future brain-boosting cocktail provided I knew that it had no side effects. But how would I know that? If memory pills improve working memory but at the same time reduce creativity, maybe they would be of benefit to some people with concentration difficulties but not to others. If antidepressants make us happier but eradicate our ability to fall in love, we might be heading toward a more efficient but less interesting society. This might sound obvious to those familiar with Aldous Huxley, but it is methodologically very difficult to explore the effects of, say, creativity or love, and Big Pharma has no intention of doing it for us.

It is not yet known for certain whether cognition-enhancing drugs have effects on creativity or love, but these examples have not just been plucked out of thin air. There are anecdotes about people who think that Ritalin impairs their association skills and creativity, and children who feel that the drug reduces their ability to joke around, as described in Jeffrey Zaslow's article "What if Einstein Had Taken Ritalin?"

In his book *The Man Who Mistook His Wife for a Hat*, neurologist Oliver Sacks describes a case in which a patient of his started to take a drug that worked on the dopamine system, and aside from mitigating his symptoms, it also dulled his playfulness and his creativity as a drummer. During the week, therefore, he took the medicine so he could cope with his job, but he skipped it on weekends so he could let loose on the drums with his jazz band. As regards love, it has been suggested that there are links with the serotonin system, which is the very system with which "happy pills" such as Prozac and Zoloft interact.

Improving faculties through training seems to me to be the safest way to go, but I am, of course, biased on this point, in that it is the very subject of my own research. Rather than see half the population constantly popping pills designed to boost their mental capacity, I would like to see a greater focus on mental health care in the form of mental gymnastics. Why not introduce the training of attention and working memory into the school curriculum?

Maybe we can make game companies furnish their products with a cognitive ingredients list specifying the working memory load of the games so that we can be just as informed when choosing our mental diet as we are when choosing our breakfast cereals. Instead of a glycemic index, could not some other ratio between stimulus-driven and controlled attention be worked out, or perhaps the percentage of working-memory-demanding playing time?

15 ■
The Information Flood and Flow

When you are trying to listen to the newscaster on CNN while reading the news ticker showing share prices at the bottom of the screen, your subjective feeling may well be that you are teetering on the threshold of your ability to digest information. Your brain is being inundated. If we analyze the situation through the lens of the concept of working memory, we find that your feelings are matched by something quantifiable: the simultaneous inflow of two streams of information is extremely demanding on working memory. Certain parts of your frontal and parietal lobes are imposing a limit on how much information you can assimilate. When you try to read a complicated article on the Internet while ignoring the advertisements playing out at the edge of your visual field, you are confronted with a distraction task that places a heavy load on your working memory. When you use the help function in Word, you will likely have to read each instruction several times to assimilate all the information with which your working memory is being overburdened.

Many changes in the information society that are somewhat loosely termed "greater complexity" or "higher information flow" can be traced back to an increase in working memory load. We have witnessed an accelerating rate of change in recent years, and there is no sign of it slowing down. Mobile technology is increasing the number of situations in which we try to dual-task, and cell phone conversations are probably just the beginning. Wireless communication and laptop computers will create an abundance of new simultaneous situations. With portable computers and Wi-Fi, we will see just as much Internet surfing on the streets and in cafés as we do cell phone use. Automobile GPS devices are becoming increasingly popular, and I look forward with great anticipation to the first studies showing how much delay in reaction times they cause. Some futuristic ideas, such as screens built into glasses, are already becoming a reality.

In an environment with a higher degree of distraction and heavier information demands, we often have the feeling of being distracted and unfocused, in the very same way as described in the introduction to illustrate the nature of the modern office. It is easy to connect the dots and come up with the picture that these greater cognitive demands have a damaging effect on our brain. There is, fortunately, no research suggesting that exposure to mentally more demanding or challenging situations impairs our powers of concentration. Indeed, there is much that points to the contrary: it is in situations that push the boundaries of our abilities that we train our brains the most. An interpretation of the Flynn effect is that it is these very demands and the greater complexity of our lives that make us progressively better at handling information and solving problems.

Instead, a possible reason why we feel a lack of focus is related to the discrepancy between demand and capacity. In other words, what we experience is a *relative* attention-deficit. The mechanism at work is the same as with ADHD, where the balance between challenge and skill is not maintained. Looking at the situation of the man in the street, we see that instead of diminishing his abilities, information load places extra weight on the demands he faces. You are very possibly 10 percent better at talking on the phone while erasing spam today than you were three years ago. On the other hand, the number of e-mails you receive per day has probably shot up by 200 percent. There is, therefore, no contradiction between the feeling that your abilities are inadequate and the improvement of these abilities.

◼ Infostress

Are we to unconditionally accept the information flood in the hope that in doing so we will be developing our faculties? No, not necessarily. We must always be aware of the limited scope we have for receiving information. A concrete example of what happens when demands exceed capacity is cell-phone-related road accidents.

The other factor telling us that we ought to embrace the burgeoning information flood with certain reservations is the link it has with stress. Our understanding of stress has deepened over the years, and there are countless studies showing how high levels of stress hormones damage the heart, the blood vessels, the immune system, and almost every other part of the body, including the brain. As regards this last organ, we can link increased stress with impaired working memory and impaired long-term memory. Scientists have also shown that stress, particularly of the severe kind, such as post-traumatic stress, affects the hippocampus, a brain structure important to the storing of information in long-term memory. But this applies to prolonged, high levels of stress; moderate, temporary stress can be a good thing and, like arousal, has an optimal level of effect (see page 22).

Nor is there any simple connection between volume of information and stress hormones. In *Why Zebras Don't Get Ulcers*, Robert Sapolsky reviews his and other people's research into stress and its underlying factors. Levels of stress are contextual and related to our interpretation of the situations in which we find ourselves. A key concept is *sense of control*. Stress is primarily associated with situations that we either feel or know we cannot control. "Learned helplessness" is a term coined to describe those who have learned that they are powerless to influence their situation. Stress is therefore very much a matter of our own attitude. Technological problems that cause certain people to break out in a cold sweat are to others nothing but entertaining challenges.

One study has documented how people perceive their e-mail burden. It turns out that most people claim that they receive too many e-mails, bordering on the limits of their ability to cope. What is interesting, though, is that the extent to which they complained was totally independent of the number of e-mails they received. Those who received twenty a day protested just as much as those who received a hundred. If we associate information load with entertaining challenges and the development of our capacity, might our infostress decrease?

■ Why We Love Stimulation

Exceeding the limits of our capacity rarely brings success. However, this does not mean that we are to keep as far away from it as we can. There is also an interesting tendency for us to push our own boundaries. We want more information, more impressions, and more complexity. Game development is an example of this. The latest incarnation of Nintendo's Game Boy console, which is mainly targeted at younger users, has two screens designed to be played upon simultaneously. We will have to assume that Nintendo has done its homework thoroughly and found that this simultaneous situation is something that appeals to children and teenagers. Similarly, the games themselves are becoming all the more complex.

Many people seek out situations that demand concurrent performance or situations in which they are overwhelmed with information. When someone takes out a cell phone during a meeting to send a text message or read e-mails, it is a voluntary action and not something that makes them simply victims of ruthless technological progress. Steven Johnson has shown how TV programs are becoming ever more complex rather than less so, their multiple interwoven plot lines demanding more and more from us in terms of problem solving if we are to have any chance of understanding the narrative development. There is clearly something inherently attractive about programs that are more complex. Johnson also argues that the more complicated computer programs fulfill a need within us to probe and seek stimulation.

◼ Flow

The American psychologist Mihály Csíkszentmihályi has written about the concept of *flow*, which is the feeling we have of being completely focused on and absorbed in the work we are doing. An artist painting a picture who is so engrossed in his work that he becomes unaware of himself and the passage of time is in a state of flow. Flow can also be attained when a surgeon performs a difficult operation in which she has to use all her abilities and skills. What Csíkszentmihályi has tried to do is identify the circumstances that elicit flow. He reasons that if we analyze situations in terms of the challenges they present and the skills of the person involved in them, we find that flow arises in

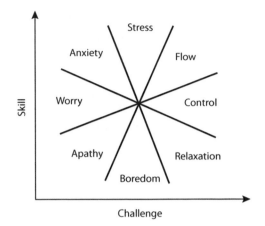

FIGURE 15-1
Csíkszentmihályi's map of how different mental states can be conceived as
a product of challenge and skill (adapted from Csíkszentmihályi, 1997).

contexts characterized by a high level of challenge and
skill, in which the capacity of the doer exactly matches the
demands of the task being done.

Considering Csíkszentmihályi's diagram as a cognitive
map with north at the top, it is in the northeast sector
where we find the state of flow. When challenge exceeds
skill, we get stress. When skill exceeds challenge, we get a
sense of control, which becomes boredom as the level of
challenge drops. Exchange "skill" for "working memory
capacity" and "challenge" for "information load," and perhaps we have a map illustrating the subjective side of the
information demand. When this demand exceeds our capacity, we experience the relative attention deficit due north
on the map. However, we should not simply avoid these
demands, for when they are too low we become bored and
apathetic. In other words, there is a reason for us to cater to
our need for stimulation and information. It is when demand
and capacity, or skill and challenge, are in a state of equilib-
rium that the situation is conducive to flow. And perhaps it

is precisely here, where we exploit our full capacity, that we develop and train our abilities.

When working memory load exactly matches working memory capacity and we hover around the magical number seven, the training effect is its most powerful. Now that we know this, it is up to us to control our environments and reshape the work we do to our abilities. Let us hope that we can learn to perfect the compass that will show us where to find balance and help us navigate into the northeastern corner of the map, where we can feel flow and develop to our full capacity.

Notes and References ■

CHAPTER 1: INTRODUCTION: THE STONE AGE BRAIN MEETS
THE INFORMATION FLOOD

4 Studies on distractions at the workplace are described in C. Thompson, "Meet the Life Hackers," *New York Times*, October 16, 2005. One of Hallowell's works on attention deficit trait is E. Hallowell, "Overloaded Circuits: Why Smart People Underperform," *Harvard Business Review*, January 2005.

7 Miller's speech on the magical number seven: G. A. Miller, "The Magical Number Seven, Plus or Minus Two: Some Limits on Our Capacity for Processing Information," *Psychological Review* 63 (1956): 81–97.

11 The plasticity of the somatosensory areas is described in J. H. Kaas, M. M. Merzenich, and H. P. Killackey, "The Reorganization of Somatosensory Cortex Following Peripheral Nerve Damage in Adult and Developing Mammals," *Annual Review of Neuroscience* 6 (1983): 325–56; J. H. Kaas, "Plasticity of Sensory and Motor Maps

in Adult Mammals," *Annual Review of Neuroscience* 14 (1991): 137–67.

12   The visual cortices of blind people: N. Sadato, A. Pascual-Leone, J. Grafman, et al., "Activation of the Primary Visual Cortex by Braille Reading in Blind Subjects," *Nature* 380 (1996): 526–28.

12   The auditory cortices of deaf people: L. A. Petitto, R. J. Zatorre, K. Gauna, et al., "Speech-like Cerebral Activity in Profoundly Deaf People Processing Signed Languages: Implications for the Neural Basis of Human Language," *Proceedings of the National Academy of Science of the United States of America* 97 (2000): 13961–66.

12   Brain differences in string musicians: T. Elbert, C. Pantev, C. Wienbruch, et al., "Increased Cortical Representation of the Fingers of the Left Hand in String Players," *Science* 270 (1995): 305–7.

12   Brain activity and piano notes: C. Pantev, R. Oostenveld, A. Engelien, et al., "Increased Auditory Cortical Representation in Musicians," *Nature* 392 (1998): 811–14.

12   Pathways in musicians: S. L. Bengtsson, Z. Nagy, S. Skare, et al., "Extensive Piano Practicing Has Regionally Specific Effects on White Matter Development," *Nature Neuroscience* 8 (2005): 1148–50.

12   Juggling: B. Draganski, C. Gaser, V. Busch, et al., "Neuroplasticity: Changes in Grey Matter Induced by Training," *Nature* 427 (2004): 311–12.

13   The Flynn effect is described in a number of publications, including J. Flynn, "Massive Gains in 14 Nations: What IQ Tests Really Measure," *Psychological Bulletin* 101 (1987): 171–91, and J. Flynn, "Searching for Justice: The Discovery of IQ Gains over Time," *American Psychologist* 54 (1999): 5–20.

16   The article on neurocognitive enhancement: M. J. Farah, J. Illes, R. Cook-Deegan, et al., "Neurocognitive Enhancement: What Can We Do and What Should We Do?" *Nature Reviews Neuroscience* 5 (2004): 421–25.

21   There are many models of attention, and with about
      fifteen hundred new articles coming out each year on the
      subject, there is no consensus about how to differentiate
      between types of attention. The model given here is
      based on recent studies of brain activity during different
      kinds of attention task. For a summary of these studies,
      see M. Corbetta and G. L. Shulman, "Control of Goal-
      Directed and Stimulus-Driven Attention in the Brain,"
      Nature Reviews Neuroscience 3 (2002): 201–15, and S.
      Kastner and L. G. Ungerleider, "Mechanisms of Visual
      Attention in the Human Cortex," *Annual Reviews of
      Neuroscience* 23 (2000): 315–41.

      The model is largely based on Michael Posner's
      measurements of different kinds of attention, as described
      in M. I. Posner, *Chronometric Explorations of Mind*
      (Hillsdale, N.J.: Erlbaum, 1978), and M. I. Posner,
      "Orienting of Attention," *Quarterly Journal of Experimental
      Psychology* 32 (1980): 3–25.

      Michael Posner uses the term *orientation* to describe
      selective attention. He also discusses another form of
      attention, which he called *executive attention*; see
      M. I. Posner and S. E. Petersen, "The Attention System
      of the Human Brain," *Annual Review of Neuroscience* 13
      (1990): 25–42. Examples of tasks that engage this type of
      attention are the Stroop and Ericson Flanker tasks.
      However, these tasks are often classified as inhibition
      tasks and will not be dealt with here. There are several
      synonyms for controlled and stimulus-driven attention,
      such as "top-down" and "bottom-up" attention, or
      "endogenous" and "exogenous" attention.

21   Arousal: J. F. Mackworth, *Vigilance and Attention*
      (Baltimore: Penguin, 1970).

22   The violinist anecdote is taken from D. L. Schacter, *The
      Seven Sins of Memory: How the Mind Forgets and Remembers*
      (New York: Houghton Mifflin, 2001).

23   Posner's studies: M. I. Posner, *Chronometric Explorations of
      Mind* (Hillsdale, N.J.: Erlbaum, 1978), and M. I. Posner,

"Orienting of Attention," *Quarterly Journal of Experimental Psychology* 32 (1980): 3–25.

24   The relationship between different kinds of attention: J. Fan, B. D. McCandliss, T. Sommer, et al., "Testing the Efficiency and Independence of Attentional Networks," *Journal of Cognitive Neuroscience* 14 (2002): 340–47.

24   The computer game and ADHD study: V. Lawrence, S. Houghton, R. Tannock, et al., "ADHD Outside the Laboratory: Boys' Executive Function Performance on Tasks in Videogame Play and on a Visit to the Zoo," *Journal of Abnormal Child Psychology* 30 (2002): 447–62.

26   fMRI study of attention: J. A. Brefczynski and E. A. DeYoe, "A Physiological Correlate of the 'Spotlight' of Visual Attention," *Nature Neuroscience* 2 (1999): 370–74. The "spotlight" analogy for attention has been drawn by other scientists, including F. Sengpiel and M. Hubener, "Visual Attention: Spotlight on the Primary Visual Cortex," *Current Biology* 9 (1999): R318–21. More recent studies have shown that the neurons not only increase their response rate when a stimulus appears; it also seems as if the neurons of a particular area become more synchronized by attention (i.e., different neurons are activated simultaneously). The rhythm is extremely fast, between 40 and 70 oscillations per second. Measurements of the synchronicity of nerve cells before a stimulus appears even make it possible to predict how quick the reaction will be. See T. Womelsdorf, P. Fries, P. P. Mitra, et al., "Gammaband Synchronization in Visual Cortex Predicts Speed of Change Detection," *Nature* 439 (2006): 733–36.

27   For early studies of attention and the sense of touch, see P. E. Roland, "Somatotopical Tuning of the Postcentral Gyrus During Focal Attention in Man. A Regional Cerebral Blood Flow Study," *Journal of Neurophysiology* 46 (1981): 744–54, and P. E. Roland, "Cortical Regulation of Selective Attention in Man. A Regional Cerebral Blood Flow Study," *Journal of Neurophysiology* 48 (1982): 1959–78.

27   The study of competition between neurons: B. C. Motter, "Focal Attention Produces Spatially Selective Processing in Visual Cortical Areas V1, V2, and V4 in the Presence of

Competing Stimuli," *Journal of Neurophysiology* 70 (1993): 909–19.

29   Evidence for different systems of attention is summarized in M. Corbetta and G. L. Shulman, "Control of Goal-Directed and Stimulus-Driven Attention in the Brain," *Nature Reviews Neuroscience* 3 (2002): 201–15. Original studies include S. Kastner, M. A. Pinsk, P. De Weerd, et al., "Increased Activity in Human Visual Cortex During Directed Attention in the Absence of Visual Stimulation," *Neuron* 22 (1999): 751–61, and J. B. Hopfinger, M. H. Buonocore, and G. R. Mangun, "The Neural Mechanisms of Top-Down Attentional Control," *Nature Neuroscience* 3 (2000): 284–91. Illustration adapted from Corbetta and Shulman, "Control of Goal-Directed and Stimulus-Driven Attention in the Brain." It should be pointed out that the frontal and parietal cortices are not the only areas connected with selective attention. David LeBerge and others have ascribed a critical role to a group of nerve cells in the brain stem called the colliculus superior, which seems to contain a spatial map of an individual's surroundings and which connects to the areas of the neocortex. Another structure of possible importance to attention is the thalamus, a cluster of neurons in the middle of the brain consisting of a large number of nuclei, such as the pulvinar nucleus and the reticular nucleus. These nuclei are connected to large areas of the neocortex and are therefore well placed to convey attention. Francis Crick, who was awarded the Nobel prize for the discovery of the structure of DNA, decided later in life to change his field of research to the brain, in particular the problem of the origin of consciousness. (He was not known for his humility, and was said to have upbraided someone who introduced him as the winner of a Nobel prize: "Not a Nobel prize, *the* Nobel prize.") In 1984 he wrote an article entitled "Functions of the Thalamic Reticular Complex: The Searchlight Hypothesis," in which he makes a case for the role played by the reticular nucleus in the context and likens attention to a light beam. Function of the thalamic reticular complex: the searchlight hypothesis. Proc Natl Acad Sci U S A. 1984 Jul;81(14):4586–90.

31   Neglect: M. Gazzaniga, R. B. Ivry, and G. R. Mangun,
       Cognitive Neuroscience, 2nd ed. (New York: Norton,
       2002).

CHAPTER 3: THE MENTAL WORKBENCH

34   Original description of working memory: K. Pribram, in
       G. A. Miller, E. Galanter, and K. H. Pribram, eds., *Plans
       and the Structure of Behavior* (New York: Holt, 1960).

34   Model of working memory: A. D. Baddeley and G. J.
       Hitch, "Working Memory," in G. A. Bower, ed., *Recent
       Advances in Learning and Motivation*, vol. 8 (New York:
       Academic Press, 1974), 47–89. A more recent account
       appears in A. Baddeley, "Working Memory: Looking Back
       and Looking Forward," *Nature Reviews Neuroscience* 4
       (2003): 829–39.

36   On the effects of electroconvulsive therapy on long-term
       memory, see L. R. Squire, *Memory and Brain* (New York:
       Oxford University Press, 1987).

40   The term "attentional template" was coined in R. Desimone
       and J. Duncan, "Neural Mechanisms of Selective Visual
       Attention," *Annual Reviews of Neuroscience* 18 (1995):
       193–222. For an account of the overlap between working
       memory and attention, see R. Desimone, "Neural
       Mechanisms for Visual Memory and Their Role in
       Attention," *Proceedings of the National Academy of Sciences
       of the United States of America* 93 (1996): 13494–99, and E.
       Awh and J. Jonides, "Overlapping Mechanisms of
       Attention and Spatial Working Memory," *Trends in
       Cognitive Sciences* 5 (2001): 119–26.

41   Quote from A. Baddeley, "Working Memory," *Science* 255
       (1992): 556–59. The example of a Raven's matrix given
       here is not one of the tasks published in the original tests,
       which are copyrighted, but is constructed along similar
       lines. Original Raven's matrices can be found in J. C.
       Raven, *Advanced Progressive Matrices: Set II* (Oxford:
       Oxford Psychology Press, 1990).

42   Article on working memory and reasoning: P. C.
       Kyllonen and R. E. Christal, "Reasoning Ability Is (Little

More than) Working-Memory Capacity?!," *Intelligence* 14 (1990): 389–433. Quote from H.-M. Süß, K. Oberauer, W. W. Wittmann, et al., "Working-Memory Capacity Explains Reasoning Ability—and a Little Bit More," *Intelligence* 20 (2002): 261–88.

42 Studies of working memory and gF: R. W. Engle, M. J. Kane, and S. W. Tuholski, "Individual Differences in Working-Memory Capacity and What They Tell Us About Controlled Attention, General Fluid Intelligence and Functions of the Prefrontal Cortex," in A. Shah and P. Shah, eds., *Models of Working Memory: Mechanisms of Active Maintenance and Executive Control*, 102–34 (New York: Cambridge University Press, 1999). Engle found higher correlations for more complex working memory tasks (such as reading span, which is partly a simultaneous task) than for simple verbal working memory tasks involving recognizing or repeating spoken words. One problem with Engle's studies is that they included only verbal tasks. Simple visuospatial working memory tasks have just as high a degree of correlation with Raven's matrices as the complex verbal tasks used by Engle. See, for example, K. Oberauer, H.-M. Süß, O. Wilhelm, et al., "Individual Differences in Working Memory Capacity and Reasoning Ability," in R. A. Conway, C. Jarrold, M. J. Kane, et al., eds., *Variation in Working Memory* (New York: Oxford University Press, 2007). For a discussion and more examples, see T. Klingberg, "Development of a Superior Frontal-Intraparietal Network for Visuo-Spatial Working Memory," *Neuropsychologia* 44, 11(2006): 2171–77; A. F. Fry and S. Hale, "Relationships Among Processing Speed, Working Memory, and Fluid Intelligence in Children," *Biological Psychology* 54 (2000): 1–34; and H.-M. Süß, K. Oberauer, W. W. Wittmann, et al., "Working-memory Capacity Explains Reasoning Ability—and a Little Bit More," *Intelligence* 30, 3 (2002): 261–28. A summarized account of the relation and correlation between working memory and intelligence can be found in A. R. Conway, M. J. Kane, and R. W. Engle, "Working Memory Capacity and Its Relation to General Intelligence," *Trends in Cognitive Sciences* 7 (2003): 547–52.

43   On the correlation between gF and memory tasks without manipulation, see Oberauer, Süß, Wilhelm, et al., "Individual differences in working memory capacity and reasoning ability," and N. Unsworth and R. W. Engle, "On the Division of Short-Term and Working Memory: An Examination of Simple and Complex Span and Their Relation to Higher Order Abilities," *Psychological Bulletin* 133 (2007): 1038–66.

There is an ongoing discussion on the differences in activity between various kinds of working memory task and differences between short-term memory and working memory. It has been proposed that the ventral (lower) parts of the prefrontal lobes are activated by nonmanipulative working memory tasks and that the dorsolateral parts (e.g., Brodmann area 46) are activated only when manipulation is required. This was originally posited by Michael Petrides and has certain empirical support. See A. M. Owen, A. C. Evans, and M. Petrides, "Evidence for a Two-Stage Model of Spatial Working Memory Processing Within the Lateral Frontal Cortex: A Positron Emission Tomography Study," *Cerebral Cortex* 6 (1996): 31–38, and M. D'Esposito, G. K. Aguirre, E. Zarahn, et al., "Functional MRI Studies of Spatial and Nonspatial Working Memory," *Cognitive Brain Research* 7 (1998): 1–13.

However, there are many studies that contradict this theory and show that nonmanipulative working memory tasks such as the dot test activate the dorsolateral parts of the prefrontal lobe. See C. E. Curtis, V. Y. Rao, and M. D'Esposito, "Maintenance of Spatial and Motor Codes During Oculomotor Delayed Response Tasks," *Journal of Neuroscience* 24 (2004): 3944–52. Here it is shown that these areas are also continually active during the delay period when no manipulation is done, corroborating previous findings by, for example, J. D. Cohen, W. M. Pearstein, T. S. Braver, et al., "Temporal Dynamics of Brain Activation During a Working-Memory Task," *Nature* 386 (1997): 604–8.

D'Esposito and Curtis summarize the difference between tasks with and without manipulation thus: "The distinction between representation and operations can be made clear in the vernacular of our cognitive models, but as we shall see, it might prove extremely difficult to distinguish between them with our current indirect (e.g. fMRI) and even direct measures (e.g. unit recordings) of neuronal activity." C. E. Curtis and M. D'Esposito, "Persistent Activity in the Prefrontal Cortex During Working Memory," *Trends in Cognitive Sciences* 7 (2003): 415–23. If one wants to create a nomenclature congruent with the brain activity data, it is thus difficult to differentiate between these two categories of working memory task. I leave a more in-depth discussion on this to scientific publications on the subject.

CHAPTER 4: MODELS OF WORKING MEMORY

46   One of the most widely cited studies of neuronal activity during working memory tasks is S. Funahashi, C. J. Bruce, and P. S. Goldman-Rakic, "Mnemonic Coding of Visual Space in the Monkey's Dorsolateral Prefrontal Cortex," *Journal of Neurophysiology* 61 (1989): 331–49. The earliest study is J. M. Fuster and G. E. Alexander, "Neuron Activity Related to Short-Term Memory," *Science* 173 (1971): 652–54.

47   Computer simulations of working memory activity are reviewed, for example, in X.-J.Wang, "Synaptic Reverberation Underlying Mnemonic Persistent Activity," *Trends in Neuroscience* 24 (2001). See also J. Tegner, A. Compte, and X.-J. Wang, "The Dynamical Stability of Reverberatory Neural Circuits," *Biological Cybernetics* 87 (2002): 471–81.

48   PET studies of working memory: E. Paulesu, C. D. Frith, and R. S. J. Frackowiak, "The Neural Correlates of the Verbal Component of Working Memory," *Nature* 362 (1993): 342–45, and J. Jonides, E. E. Smith, R. A. Koeppe, et al., "Spatial Working Memory in Humans as Revealed by PET," *Nature* 363 (1993): 623–25.

49   fMRI studies showing continual activity: J. D. Cohen, W. M. Pearstein, T. S. Braver, et al., "Temporal Dynamics of Brain Activation During a Working-Memory Task,"

Nature 386 (1997), and S. M. Courtney, L. G. Ungerleider, K. Keil, et al., "Transient and Sustained Activity in a Distributed Neural System for Human Working Memory," *Nature* 386 (1997): 608–11.

49   Continual activity during the dot test: C. E. Curtis, V. Y. Rao, and M. D'Esposito, "Maintenance of Spatial and Motor Codes During Oculomotor Delayed Response Tasks," *Journal of Neuroscience* 24 (2004): 3944–52.

51   Illustration adapted from C. E. Curtis and M. D'Esposito, "Persistent Activity in the Prefrontal Cortex During Working Memory," *Trends in Cognitive Sciences* 7 (2003): 415–23.

51   Studies supporting the specialized neuron theory: S. Funahashi, C. J. Bruce, and P. S. Goldman-Rakic, "Mnemonic Coding of Visual Space in the Monkey's Dorsolateral Prefrontal Cortex," *Journal of Neurophysiology* 61 (1989): 331–49.

51   Studies supporting the multimodal cell theory: J. Quintana and J. M. Fuster, "Mnemonic and Predictive Functions of Cortical Neurons in a Memory Task," *Neuroreport* 3 (1992): 721–24. For a review, see J. M. Fuster, *Memory in the Cerebral Cortex* (Cambridge, Mass.: MIT Press, 1995).

52   The theory of parallel working-memory systems: P. S. Goldman-Rakic, "Topography of Cognition: Parallel Distributed Networks in Primate Association Cortex," *Annual Reviews of Neuroscience* 11 (1988): 137–56.

52   Studies of multimodal areas: T. Klingberg, P. E. Roland, and R. Kawashima, "Activation of Multi-modal Cortical Areas Underlies Short-Term Memory," *European Journal of Neuroscience* 8 (1996): 1965–71, and T. Klingberg, "Concurrent Performance of Two Working-Memory Tasks: Potential Mechanisms of Interference," *Cerebral Cortex* 8 (1998): 593–601.

52   Examples of other studies indicating bottlenecks and overlaps between modalities: J. Duncan and A. M. Owen, "Common Regions of the Human Frontal Lobe Recruited by Diverse Cognitive Demands," *Trends in Neurosciences* 23 (2000): 475–83; H. Hautzel, F. M. Mottaghy, D. Schmidt, et al., "Topographic Segregation and Convergence of

Verbal, Object, Shape and Spatial Working Memory in Humans," *Neuroscience Letters* 323 (2002): 156–60; and C. E. Curtis and M. D'Esposito, "Persistent Activity in the Prefrontal Cortex During Working Memory," *Trends in Cognitive Sciences* 7 (2003): 415–23.

CHAPTER 5: THE BRAIN AND THE MAGICAL NUMBER SEVEN

55   Miller's original article is G. A. Miller, "The Magical Number Seven, Plus or Minus Two: Some Limits on Our Capacity for Processing Information," *Psychological Review* 63 (1956): 81–97. See also N. Cowan, "The Magical Number 4 in Short-Term Memory: A Reconsideration of Mental Storage Capacity," *Behavioral and Brain Sciences* 24 (2001): 87–185.

57   Study of working memory in infants: A. Diamond and P. S. Goldman-Rakic, "Comparison of Human Infants and Rhesus Monkeys on Piaget's AB Task: Evidence for Dependence on Dorsolateral Prefrontal Cortex," *Experimental Brain Research* 74, 1 (1989): 24–40.

58   Studies of the development of working memory: S. E. Gathercole, S. J. Pickering, B. Ambridge, et al., "The Structure of Working Memory from 4 to 15 Years of Age," *Developmental Psychology* 40 (2004): 177–90; S. Hale, M. D. Bronik, and A. F. Fry, "Verbal and Spatial Working Memory in School-Age Children: Developmental Differences in Susceptibility to Interference," *Developmental Psychology* 33 (1997): 364–71; and H. Westerberg, T. Hirvikoski, H. Forssberg, et al., "Visuospatial Working Memory: A Sensitive Measurement of Cognitive Deficits in ADHD," *Child Neuropsychology* 10 (2004): 155–61.

58   On working memory and problem-solving skills in children: A. F. Fry and S. Hale, "Processing Speed, Working Memory, and Fluid Intelligence," *Psychological Science* 7 (1996): 237–41.

58   Fig. 5.1. Data for the graph of working memory and age were taken from H. L. Swanson, "What Develops in Working Memory? A Life Span Perspective," *Developmental Psychology* 35 (1999): 986–1000.

59 Studies of the game of Concentration in children and adults: L. Baker-Ward and P. A. Ornstein, "Age Differences in Visual-Spatial Memory Performance: Do Children Really Out-perform Adults When Playing Concentration?" *Bulletin of the Psychonomic Society* 26 (1988): 331–32, and M. Gulya, A. Rosse-George, K. Hartshorn, et al., "The Development of Explicit Memory for Basic Perceptual Feature," *Journal of Experimental Child Psychology* 81 (2002): 276–97.

60 Changes in brain activity during childhood: T. Klingberg, H. Forssberg, and H. Westerberg, "Increased Brain Activity in Frontal and Parietal Cortex Underlies the Development of Visuo-spatial Working Memory Capacity During Childhood," *Journal of Cognitive Neuroscience* 14 (2002): 1–10. Studies containing measurements of brain activity and myelinization: P. J. Olesen, Z. Nagy, H. Westerberg, et al., "Combined Analysis of DTI and fMRI Data Reveals a Joint Maturation of White and Grey Matter in a Fronto-parietal Network," *Cognitive Brain Research* 18 (2003): 48–57. One study that also includes distraction during the working memory task is P. Olesen, J. Macoveanu, J. Tegner, et al., "Brain Activity Related Working Memory and Distraction in Children and Adults," *Cerebral Cortex*, June 26, 2006 (e-pub ahead of print).

60 Other studies on the development of visuospatial memory confirming these results: H. Kwon, A. L. Reiss, and V. Menon, "Neural Basis of Protracted Developmental Changes in Visuo-spatial Working Memory," *Proceedings of the National Academy of Sciences USA* 99 (2002): 13336–41.

61 fMRI study of capacity and the parietal lobe: J. J. Toddand R. Marois, "Capacity Limit of Visual Short-Term Memory in Human Posterior Parietal Cortex," *Nature* 428 (2004): 751–54. EEG study giving similar results: E. K. Vogel and M. G. Machizawa, "Neural Activity Predicts Individual Differences in Visual Working Memory Capacity," *Nature* 428 (2004): 748–51.

61 Correlation between performance on Raven's matrices and brain activity: K. H. Lee, Y. Y. Choi, J. R. Gray, et al., "Neural Correlates of Superior Intelligence: Stronger

Recruitment of Posterior Parietal Cortex," *Neuroimage* 29 (2006): 578–86. A correlation between performance on Raven's matrices and frontal and parietal activity when people are performing working memory tasks has also been shown by J. R. Gray, C. F. Chabris, and T. S. Braver, "Neural Mechanisms of General Fluid Intelligence," *Nature Neuroscience* 6 (2003): 316–22.

62   The study of Albert Einstein's brain: S. F. Witelson, D. L. Kigar, and T. Harvey, "The Exceptional Brain of Albert Einstein," *Lancet* 353 (1999): 2149–53.

63   Summarized account of information load and brain activity: T. Klingberg, "Limitations in Information Processing in the Human Brain: Neuroimaging of Dual Task Performance and Working Memory Tasks," *Progress in Brain Research* 126 (2000): 95–102.

64   Synaptic density and development: P. Huttenlocher, "Synaptic Density in Human Frontal Cortex— Developmental Changes and Effects of Aging," *Brain Research* 163 (1979): 195–205.

64   The loss of axons during development: A. S. LaMantia and P. Rakic, "Axon Overproduction and Elimination in the Corpus Callosum of the Developing Rhesus Monkey," *Journal of Neuroscience* 10 (1990): 2156–75.

64   Histological studies of myelinization: P. I. Yakovlev and A.-R. Lecours, "The Myelogenetic Cycles of Regional Maturation of the Brain," in A. Minkowsi, ed., *Regional Development of the Brain in Early Life*, 3–70 (Oxford: Blackwell Scientific Publications, 1967). An MR scanner can provide an indirect measure of myelinization using a technique called diffusion tensor imaging, which measures the diffusion of water in the white matter. This technique was used to study the development of white matter in Z. Nagy, H. Westerberg, and T. Klingberg, "Regional Maturation of White Matter During Childhood and Development of Function," *Journal of Cognitive Neuroscience* 16 (2004): 1227–33. In another diffusion study, myelinization was linked to changes in brain activity: Olesen, Nagy, Westerberg, et al., "Combined analysis of DTI and fMRI data."

66   Modeling of neuronal activity: F. Edin, J. Macoveanu,
      P. Olesen, et al., "Stronger Synaptic Connectivity as a
      Mechanism Behind Development of Working Memory–
      Related Brain Activity During Childhood," *Journal of
      Cognitive Neuroscience* 19 (2007): 750–60.

CHAPTER 6: SIMULTANEOUS CAPACITY AND MENTAL BANDWIDTH

70   Fig. 6.1.Graph adapted from M. Posner, *Chronometric
      Explorations of Mind* (Hillsdale, N.J.: Erlbaum, 1978).

71   On sex differences in dual-task ability: M. Hiscock,
      N. Perachio, and R. Inch, "Is There a Sex Difference in
      Human Laterality? IV. An Exhaustive Survey of
      Dual-Task Interference Studies from Six Neuropsychology
      Journals," *Journal of Clinical and Experimental
      Neuropsychology* 23 (2001): 137–48.

72   Studies of concurrent performance: D. L. Strayer and
      W. A. Johnston, "Driven to Distraction: Dual-Task Studies
      of Simulated Driving and Conversing on a Cellular
      Telephone," *Psychological Science* 12 (2001): 462–66.
      Estimates of deaths: "How Many Things Can You
      Do at Once," *New Scientist*, April 7, 2007. H. Alm and
      L. Nilsson, "The Effects of a Mobile Telephone Task on
      Driver Behaviour in a Car Following Situation," *Accident
      Analysis and Prevention* 27 (1995): 707–15.

73   On working memory and distraction: N. Lavie, A. Hirst,
      J. W. de Fockert, et al., "Load Theory of Selective
      Attention and Cognitive Control," *Journal of Experimental
      Psychology* 133 (2004): 339–54. A summarized account is in
      N. Lavie, "Distracted and Confused? Selective Attention
      Under Load," *Trends in Cognitive Sciences* 9 (2005): 75–82.
      Brain activity during distraction is reported in J. W. de
      Fockert, G. Rees, C. D. Frith, et al., "The Role of Working
      Memory in Visual Selective Attention," *Science* 291 (2001):
      1803–6.

73   On working memory capacity and distractibility:
      E. K. Vogel, A. W. McCollough, and M. G. Machizawa,
      "Neural Measures Reveal Individual Differences in
      Controlling Access to Working Memory," *Nature* 438

(2005): 500–3. On the control of filtering: F. McNab and T. Klingberg, "Prefrontal Cortex and Basal Ganglia Control Access to Working Memory," *Nature Neuroscience* 11, 1 (2008): 103–7.

75 Working memory capacity and the cocktail party effect: A. R. Conway, N. Cowan, and M. F. Bunting, "The Cocktail Party Phenomenon Revisited: The Importance of Working Memory Capacity," *Psychonomic Bulletin amd Review* 8 (2001): 331–35.

75 Study of mind-wandering: M. J. Kane, L. H. Brown, J. C. McVay et al. "For whom the mind wanders, and when. An experience-sampling study of working memory and executive control in daily life." *Psychological Science* 18 (2007) 614–21.

77 fMRI study of the central executive: M. D'Esposito, J. A. Detre, D. C. Alsop, et al., "The Neural Basis of the Central Executive System of Working Memory," *Nature* 378 (1995): 279–81.

78 Studies of the alternative hypothesis of interference during concurrent performance: T. Klingberg and P. E. Roland, "Interference Between Two Concurrent Tasks Is Associated with Activation of Overlapping Fields in the Cortex," *Cognitive Brain Research* 6 (1997): 1–8; T. Klingberg, "Concurrent Performance of Two Working Memory Tasks: Potential Mechanisms of Interference," *Cerebral Cortex* 8 (1998); and T. Klingberg, "Limitations in Information Processing in the Human Brain: Neuroimaging of Dual Task Performance and Working Memory Tasks," *Progress in Brain Research* 126 (2000).

79 fMRI study of concurrent performance: S. Bunge, T. Klingberg, R. B. Jacobsen, et al., "A Resource Model of the Neural Substrates of Executive Working Memory in Humans," *Proceedings of the National Academy of Sciences USA* 97 (2000): 3573–78.

79 A study that did not manage to replicate D'Esposito's results on a separate "concurrent performance" area is R. A. Adcock, R. T. Constable, J. C. Gore, et al., "Functional Neuroanatomy of Executive Processes

Involved in Dual-Task Performance," *Proceedings of the National Academy of Sciences USA* 97 (2000): 3567–72.

79 A study that found brain activity specific to concurrent performance: E. Koechlin, G. Basso, P. Pietrini, et al., "The Role of the Anterior Prefrontal Cortex in Human Cognition," *Nature* 399 (1999): 148–51.

CHAPTER 7: WALLACE'S PARADOX

84 Quote from S. J. Gould, *The Panda's Thumb: More Reflections in Natural History* (New York: Norton, 1980), 55.

85 Fig. 7.1: Graph adapted from R. I. M. Dunbar, *Grooming, Gossip and the Evolution of Language* (London: Faber, 1996). It should be pointed out that genetic mutations occur all the time and that evolution is not something that came to a halt a few thousand years ago. Geneticists have discovered several genetic changes that have been occurring since the appearance of *Homo sapiens* 200,000 years ago. Bruce Lahn, for instance, and his team at the University of Chicago have identified two gene variants, one of which is thought to have occurred 40,000 years ago and the other only 6,000 years ago: P. D. Evans, S. L. Gilbert, N. Mekel-Bobrov, et al., "Microcephalin, a Gene Regulating Brain Size, Continues to Evolve Adaptively in Humans," *Science* 309 (2005): 1717–20, and N. Mekel Bobrov, S. L. Gilbert, P. D. Evans, et al., "Ongoing Adaptive Evolution of ASPM, a Brain Size Determinant in *Homo sapiens*," *Science* 309 (2005): 1720–22. Gene variants can be interesting, since mutations that make the gene dysfunctional lead to microcephaly, a condition whereby a baby is born with a brain around one-third of the size of a normal brain. Just what effect these gene variants have (if any) remains something of a mystery. There is no clear function for the different variants and, moreover, they appeared after the migration from Africa, meaning that they do not affect the whole of mankind. A later study also failed to find any correlation between intelligence and normal variability in this gene: N. Mekel-Bobrov et al., "The Ongoing Adaptive Evolution of ASPM and

Microcephalin Is Not Explained by Increased Intelligence," *Human Molecular Genetics* 16 (2007): 600–608.

86 Size of cortex and group size: R. I. M. Dunbar, *Grooming, Gossip and the Evolution of Language* (London: Faber, 1996).

86 Machiavellian intelligence: R. W. Byrne and A. Whiten, *Machiavellian Intelligence: Social Expertise and the Evolution of Intellect in Monkeys, Apes and Humans* (Oxford: Oxford Science Publications, 1988).

87 The role of language in the evolution of the brain: T. W. Deacon, *The Symbolic Species: The Co-evolution of Language and the Human Brain* (London: Allen Lane, 1997).

88 Evolution of intelligence and sexual selection: G. Miller, *The Mating Mind: How Sexual Choice Shaped the Evolution of Human Nature* (London: Heinemann, 2000).

89 A summarized account of Gould's arguments and his denunciation of Steven Pinker can be found in S. J. Gould, "Darwinian Fundamentalism," *New York Review of Books*, June 10, 1997, 1244. See also S. J. Gould, *The Panda's Thumb: More Reflections in Natural History* (New York: Norton, 1980), 55.

CHAPTER 8: BRAIN PLASTICITY

93 On phrenology: V. Mountcastle, "The Evolution of Ideas Concerning the Function of the Neocortex," *Cerebral Cortex* 5 (1995): 289–95.

95 Fig. 8.1a: Phrenology picture © 2002 Topham Picturepoint. Diagram of histological areas taken from K. Brodmann, *Vergleichende Lokalisationslehre der Grosshirnrinde* (Leipzig: Barth, 1909).

95 The plasticity of the somatosensory areas is described in J. H. Kaas, M. M. Merzenich, and H. P. Killackey, "The Reorganization of Somatosensory Cortex Following Peripheral Nerve Damage in Adult and Developing Mammals," *Annual Review of Neuroscience* 6 (1983): 325–56, and J. H. Kaas, "Plasticity of Sensory and Motor

Maps in Adult Mammals," *Annual Review of Neuroscience* 14 (1991): 137–67.

97 The transplantation of the visual nerve: J. Sharma, A. Angelucci, and M. Sur, "Induction of Visual Orientation Modules in Auditory Cortex," *Nature* 404 (2000): 841–47. An account of behavioral effects can be found in L. von Melchner, S. L. Pallas, and M. Sur, "Visual Behaviour Mediated by Retinal Projections Directed to the Auditory Pathway," *Nature* 404 (2000): 871–76.

98 Training and its effect on the auditory area: G. H. Recanzone, C. E. Schreiner, and M. M. Merzenich, "Plasticity in the Frequency Representation of Primary Auditory Cortex Following Discrimination Training in Adult Owl Monkeys," *Journal of Neuroscience* 13 (1993): 87–103.

98 On forelimb training and its effect on the neocortex: R. J. Nudo, G. W. Milliken, W. M. Jenkins, et al., "Use-Dependent Alterations of Movement Representations in Primary Otor Cortex of Adult Squirrel Monkeys," *Journal of Neuroscience* 16 (1996): 785–807.

98 Study of string musicians: T. Elbert, C. Pantev, C. Wienbruch, et al., "Increased Cortical Representation of the Fingers of the Left Hand in String Players," *Science* 270 (1995).

98 Study of the white matter in pianists: S. L. Bengtsson, Z. Nagy, S. Skare, et al., "Extensive Piano Practicing Has Regionally Specific Effects on White Matter Development," *Nature Neuroscience* 8 (2005).

99 fMRI study of learning finger movements: A. Karni, G. Meyer, P. Jezzard, et al., "Functional MRI Evidence for Adult Motor Cortex Plasticity During Motor Skill Learning," *Nature* 377 (1995): 155–58.

99 Juggling: B. Draganski, C. Gaser, V. Busch, et al., "Neuroplasticity: Changes in Grey Matter Induced by Training," *Nature* 427 (2004): 311–12.

Chapter 9: Does ADHD Exist?

105   Definition of ADHD: American Psychiatric Association, *Diagnostic and Statistical Manual of Mental Disorders*, 4th ed. (Washington, D.C.: American Psychiatric Association, 1994). For a review of ADHD, see J. Biederman and S. V. Faraone, "Attention-Deficit Hyperactivity Disorder," *Lancet* 366 (2005): 237–48.

109   Heredity and ADHD: Biederman and Faraone, "Attention Deficit Hyperactivity Disorder." *Lancet* 366 (2005): 237–48.

109   Hypothesis on ADHD and working memory: R. A. Barkley, "Behavioral Inhibition, Sustained Attention, and Executive Functions: Constructing a Unifying Theory of ADHD," *Psychological Bulletin* 121 (1997): 65–94.

110   Studies showing impaired working memory in cases of ADHD: J. H. Dowson, A. McLean, E. Bazanis, et al., "Impaired Spatial Working Memory in Adults with Attention-Deficit/Hyperactivity Disorder: Comparisons with Performance in Adults with Borderline Personality Disorder and in Control Subjects," *Acta Psychiatrica Scandinavica* 110 (2004): 45–54; S. Kempton, A. Vance, P. Maruff, et al., "Executive Function and Attention Deficit Hyperactivity Disorder: Stimulant Medication and Better Executive Function Performance in Children," *Psychological Medicine* 29 (1999): 527–38; and H. Westerberg, T. Hirvikoski, H. Forssberg, et al., "Visuo-spatial Working Memory: A Sensitive Measurement of Cognitive Deficits in ADHD," *Child Neuropsychology* 10 (2004): 155–61.

111   Lack of long-term effect of medication: P. S. Jensen et al., "Three-Year Follow-up of the NIMH MTA Study," *Journal of the American Academy of Child and Adolescent Psychiatry* 46 (2007): 989–1002.

112   On the effect of central stimulants on working memory: R. Barnett, P. Maruff, A. Vance, et al., "Abnormal Executive Function in Attention Deficit Hyperactivity Disorder: The Effect of Stimulant Medication and Age on Spatial Working Memory," *Psychological Medicine* 31 (2001): 1107–15, and A. C. Bedard, R. Martinussen, A. Ickowicz, et al., "Methylphenidate Improves

Visual-Spatial Memory in Children with Attention-Deficit/
Hyperactivity Disorder," *Journal of the American
Academy of Child and Adolescent Psychiatry* 43 (2004):
260–68.

112 COPE: R. A. Barkley, A. Russell, and K. R. Murphy,
Attention-Deficit Hyperactivity Disorder: A Clinical Workbook
(New York: Guilford Press, 2006).

112 TeachADHD: http://www.aboutkidshealth.ca/teachadhd.

113 Advice on ADHD: K. G. Nadeau, *ADD in the Workplace:
Choices, Changes, and Challenges* (Bristol, Penn.: Brunner/
Mazel, 1997).

Chapter 10: A Cognitive Gym

115 Earlier training studies: E. C. Butterfield, C. Wambold,
and J. M. Belmont, "On the Theory and Practice of
Improving Short-Term Memory," *American Journal of
Mental Deficiency* 77 (1973): 654–69.

116 The student who learned to memorize number series:
K. A. Ericsson, W. G. Chase, and S. Faloon, "Acquisition
of a Memory Skill," *Science* 208 (1980): 1181–82.

119 The first training study: T. Klingberg, H. Forssberg, and
H. Westerberg, "Training of Working Memory in Children
with ADHD," *Journal of Clinical and Experimental
Neuropsychology* 24 (2002): 781–91.

119 Replication of the training study involving multiple
centers: T. Klingberg, E. Fernell, P. Olesen, et al.,
"Computerized Training of Working Memory in Children
with ADHD—A Randomized, Controlled Trial," *Journal of
the American Academy of Child and Adolescent Psychiatry* 44
(2005): 177–86.

121 Other training studies: K. Dahlin, M. Myrberg,
T. Klingberg, "Training of working memory in
children with special education needs and attentional
problems" Scandinavian Journal of Psychology (in press).
American independent replications: B. Gibson et al.,
"Computerized Training of Working Memory in ADHD,"
abstract paper presented at the Conference for Children

and Adults with Attention Deficit/Hyperactivity Disorder, 2006. C. Lucas, H. Abikoff, E. Petkova, et al. "A randomized controlled trial of two forms of computerized working memory training in ADHD". Abstracted presented at American Psychiatric Association meeting, May 2008, Washington.

121   Training in healthy elderly people: H. Westerberg, Y. Brehmer, N. D'hondt, et al., "Computerized Training of Working Memory in Aging—A Controlled Randomized Trial," poster presented at the 20th Cognitive Aging Conference in Adelaide, Australia, July 12–15, 2007.

121   The clinical use and sale of the training program is the responsibility of Cogmed, a company founded and largely owned by Karolinska Development, which was established to help commercialize inventions made at Karolinska Institutet and to ensure their wider application in society. As inventors, Helena Westerberg, Jonas Beckeman, David Skoglund, and I own shares in the company but receive no royalties or similar payment based on the number of users.

122   fMRI study of working memory training: P. J. Olesen, H. Westerberg, and T. Klingberg, "Increased Prefrontal and Parietal Brain Activity After Training of Working Memory," *Nature Neuroscience* 7 (2004): 75–79.

123   Attentional process training: M. M. Sohlberg, K. A. McLaughlin, A. Pavese, et al., "Evaluation of Attention Process Training and Brain Injury Education in Persons with Acquired Brain Injury," *Journal of Clinical and Experimental Neuropsychology* 22 (2000): 656–76.

124   Other studies of working memory training: S. Jaeggi, M. Buschkuehl, J. Jonides, W.J. Perrig (2008) Improving fluid intelligence with training on working memory. *Proceedings of the National Academy of Sciences USA* 13; 105(19): 6829–33.

CHAPTER 11: THE EVERYDAY EXERCISING OF OUR MENTAL MUSCLES

127   The Einstein Aging Study: J. Verghese, R. B. Lipton, M. J. Katz, et al., "Leisure Activities and the Risk of

Dementia in the Elderly," *New England Journal of Medicine* 348 (2003): 2508–16.

128   The Stockholm (Kungsholmen) project: A. Karp, S. Paillard-Borg, H. X. Wang, et al., "Mental, Physical and Social Components in Leisure Activities Equally Contribute to Decrease Dementia Risk," *Dementia and Geriatric Cognitive Disorders* 21 (2006): 65–73. See also H. X. Wang, A. Karp, B. Winblad, et al., "Late-Life Engagement in Social and Leisure Activities Is Associated with a Decreased Risk of Dementia: A Longitudinal Study from the Kungsholmen Project," *American Journal of Epidemiology* 155 (2002): 1081–87.

130   Quote from *Dialogues of the Zen Masters*, translated into English by K. Matsuo and E. Steinilber-Oberlin, in R. P. Kapleau, *The Three Pillars of Zen* (New York: Anchor Books, 1989), 10.

132   Quote on *bompu* Zen is taken from ibid.

133   Conference on neuroscience is given in M. Barinaga, "Studying the Well- Trained Mind," *Science* 302 (2003): 44–46.

134   EEG study: A. Lutz, L. L. Greischar, N. B. Rawlings, et al., "Long-Term Meditators Self-Induce High-Amplitude Gamma Synchrony During Mental Practice," *Proceedings of the National Academy of Sciences USA* 101 (2004): 16369–73.

134   fMRI study of Buddhist monks: J. A. Brefczynski-Lewis, A. Lutz, H. S. Schaefer, et al., "Neural Correlates of Attentional Expertise in Long-Term Meditation Practitioners," *Proceeding of the National Academy of Sciences USA* 104 (2007): 11483–88.

135   Study of Zen meditators: G. Pagnoni and M. Cekic, "Age Effects on Gray Matter Volume and Attentional Performance in Zen Meditation," *Neurobiology of Aging* 28 (2007): 1623–27.

CHAPTER 12: COMPUTER GAMES

137   The story of Jennifer Grinnell comes from K. Craig, "Making a Living in Second Life," *Wired* online, February 8, 2006.

139 Quote from Tracy McVeigh, "Computer Games Stunt Teen Brains," *Observer*, August 19, 2001.

140 The positive effects of computer games: K. Durkin and B. Barber, "Not So Doomed: Computer Game Play and Positive Adolescent Development," *Journal of Applied Developmental Psychology* 23 (2002): 373–92.

141 The Tetris study: R. De Lisi and J. L. Wolford, "Improving Children's Mental Rotation Accuracy with Computer Game Playing," *Journal of Genetic Psychology* 163 (2002): 272–82.

141 Action game study: C. S. Green and D. Bavelier, "Action Video Game Modifies Visual Selective Attention," *Nature* 423 (2003): 534–37.

142 The National Institute of Public Health report: A. Lager and S. Bremberg, "Hälsoeffekter av tv- och dataspelande—en systematisk genomgång av vetenskapliga studier," National Institute of Public Health, Stockholm, 2005.

145 On Brain Age and Nintendo: I. Fuyuno, "Brain Craze," *Nature* 447 (2007): 18–20. Posit Science: H. W. Mahncke, B. B. Connor, J. Appelman, et al., "Memory Enhancement in Healthy Older Adults Using a Brain Plasticity–Based Training Program: A Randomized, Controlled Study," *Proceedings of the National Academy of Sciences USA* 103 (2006): 12523–8.

CHAPTER 13: THE FLYNN EFFECT

147 The Flynn effect is reported in, e.g., J. Flynn, "Massive Gains in 14 Nations: What IQ Tests Really Measure," *Psychological Bulletin* 101 (1987), and J. Flynn, "Searching for Justice—The Discovery of IQ Gains over Time," *American Psychologist* 54 (1999). S. Johnson "Dome improvement" Wired 13.05, May (2005).

149 Project Intelligence: R. J. Herrnstein, R. S. Nickerson, M. de Sanchez, et al., "Teaching Thinking Skills," *American Psychologist* 41 (1986): 1283.

149   The Israeli training study: R. Feuerstein, M. B. Hoffman, Y. Rand, et al., "Learning to Learn: Mediated Learning Experiences and Instrumental Enrichment," *Special Services in the Schools* 39 (1986): 49–82.

150   Kvashchev's studies: L. Stankov, "Kvashchev's Experiment: Can We Boost Intelligence?" *Intelligence* 10 (1986): 209–30.

150   Klauer's study: K. J. Klauer, K. Willmes, and G. D. Phye, "Inducing Inductive Reasoning: Does It Transfer to Fluid Intelligence?" *Contemporary Educational Psychology* 27 (2002): 1–25.

151   Effects of environment on IQ: P. M. Greenfield, "The Cultural Evolution of IQ," in U. Neisser, ed., *The Rising Curve: Long-Term Gains in IQ and Related Measures* (Washington, D.C.: American Psychological Association, 1998);

152   S. Johnson, *Everything Bad Is Good for You: How Today's Popular Culture Is Actually Making Us Smarter* (New York: Riverhead Books, 2005).

CHAPTER 14: NEUROCOGNITIVE ENHANCEMENT

157   The article on neurocognitive enhancement: M. J. Farah, J. Illes, R. Cook-Deegan, et al., "Neurocognitive Enhancement: What Can We Do and What Should We Do?" *Nature Reviews Neuroscience* 5 (2004): 421–25.

158   The effect of amphetamine on people without ADHD: J. L. Rapoport, M. S. Buchsbaum, H. Weingartner, et al., "Dextroamphetamine: Cognitive and Behavioural Effects in Normal Prepubertal Boys," *Science* 199 (1978): 560–63, J. L. Rapoport, M. S. Buchsbaum, H. Weingartner, et al., "Dextroamphetamine: Cognitive and Behavioural Effects in Normal and Hyperactive Boys and Normal Adult Males," *Archives of General Psychiatry* 37 (1980): 933–43.

158   The effects of methylphenidate (Ritalin) on people without ADHD are reported in, e.g., M. A. Mehta, A. M. Owen, B. J. Sahakian, et al., "Methylphenidate Enhances Working Memory by Modulating Discrete Frontal and Parietal Lobe Regions in the Human Brain," *Journal of Neuroscience* 20 (2000): RC65.

159   The use of central stimulants on university students is
       reported in Farah, Illes, Cook-Deegan, et al.,
       "Neurocognitive Enhancement," and Q. Babcock and
       T. Byrne, "Students' Perceptions of Methylphenidate Abuse
       at a Public Liberal Arts College," *Journal of American
       College Health* 49 (2000), and A. M. Arria K.M. Caldeira,
       K.E. O'Grady et al. "Nonmedical use of prescription
       stimulants among college students" Pharmacotherapy 28
       (2) (2008) 156–69; B. Maher. "Poll results: look who's
       doping." Nature 452 (2008) 674–75.

160   Human-computer interaction: L. R. Hochberg, M. D.
       Serruya, G. M. Friehs, et al., "Neuronal Ensemble Control
       of Prosthetic Devices by a Human with Tetraplegia,"
       Nature 442 (2006): 164–71.

161   The decrease in dopamine receptors with aging:
       L. Bäckman, N. Ginovart, R. A. Dixon, et al., "Age-Related
       Cognitive Deficits Mediated by Changes in the Striatal
       Dopamine System," *American Journal of Psychiatry* 157
       (2000): 635–37.

162   While there are anecdotal accounts of the effect of Ritalin
       and similar drugs on creativity—see, for example, J.
       Zaslow, "What if Einstein Had Taken Ritalin," *Wall Street
       Journal*, February 3, 2005, and O. Sacks, *The Man Who
       Mistook His Wife for a Hat* (London: Duckworth, 1985).
       The link between medication and creativity has not
       been demonstrated, and there are studies showing that
       Ritalin does not make children with ADHD perform
       more poorly on tests designed to measure creativity.
       See, for example, M. V. Solanto and E. H. Wender, "Does
       Methylphenidate Constrict Cognitive Functioning?"
       *Journal of the American Academy of Child and Adolescent
       Psychiatry* 28 (1989): 897–902. How Ritalin affects
       creativity in adults with ADHD, or people without
       ADHD, is unknown.

162   On serotonin and love: D. Marazziti, H. S. Akiskal,
       A. Rossi, et al., "Alteration of the Platelet Serotonin
       Transporter in Romantic Love," *Psychological Medicine* 29
       (1999): 741–45, and H. Fisher, *Why We Love: The Nature
       and Chemistry of Romantic Love* (New York: Henry Holt,
       2004).

Chapter 15: The Information Flood and Flow

166 Research on stress and its underlying factors: R. M. Sapolsky, *Why Zebras Don't Get Ulcers* (New York: W. H. Freeman, 1994).

166 The e-mail load study is from J. Glieck, *Faster: The Acceleration of Just About Everything* (London: Little, Brown, 2001).

167 On flow: M. Csíkszentmihályi, *Finding Flow: The Psychology of Engagement with Everyday Life* (New York: Basic Books, 1997).

Index ■